THE POLITICAL ECONOMY OF HEALTH
IN AFRICA

edited by

Toyin Falola

and

Dennis Ityavyar

Ohio University Center for International Studies
Monographs in International Studies

Africa Series Number 60
Athens, Ohio 1992

The books in the Center for International Studies Monograph
Series are printed on acid-free paper ∞

Library of Congress Cataloging-in-Publication Data

The Political economy of health in Africa / edited by Toyin
    Falola and Dennis Ityavyar.
        p.   cm. – (Monographs in international studies.
Africa series; no. 60)
    Includes bibliographical references.
    ISBN 0-89680-168-3
    1. Medical care–Africa. 2. Medical care–Africa–History.
3. Medical economics–Africa. 4. Medical care–Political
aspects–Africa. 5. Social medicine–Africa.
        I. Falola, Toyin. II. Ityavyar, Dennis. III. Series.
    [DNLM: 1. Delivery of Health Care–trends–Africa.
    2. Health Policy–trends–Africa. 3. Political
    systems–Africa. W 84 HA1 P7
RA418.3.A35P65   1991
362.1'096–dc20   91 - 39117
DNLM/DLIC   CIP
for Library of Congress

CONTRIBUTORS

Charles Anyinam is a medical geographer with a Ph.D. from Queen's University, Kingston, Canada. He is an assistant professor in the Department of Geography, Brock University, St. Catharines, Canada. His research interests are in traditional medicine in Ghana and primary health care in the Third World.

S. Kofi Bonsi is a Ghanaian. He obtained a B.Sc. in sociology from the University of Legon, Cape Coast, Ghana. He then obtained an M.A. at the University of Manitoba in 1971 and a Ph.D. at the University of Missouri in 1975. He is a well-known name in the sociology of medicine, and has held teaching appointments in many universities in the USA, Nigeria, and Ghana. He is now the director of the Centre for Scientific Research, Accra, Ghana.

Toyin Falola is a professor of African history at the University of Texas at Austin. Formerly he taught history at the Obafemi Awolowo University, Ile-Ife, Nigeria. He has published widely on the political economy of Africa.

U. Igun is the head of Department of Sociology at the University of Maiduguri in Nigeria. He did his B.Sc. and Ph.D. in sociology at the University of Ibadan. He has written many articles on traditional medicine.

D. A. Ityavyar obtained his B.Sc. in sociology at Ahmadu Bello University, Zaria, an M.A. from the University of Manitoba, and a Ph.D. from the University of Toronto. He has published several articles on health in Africa.

F. M. Mburu is a Kenyan. He received a B.A. degree in 1972 and an M.A. degree in 1974 in social sciences, as well as a Ph.D. in Health Care Administration from the University of Mississippi in

1976 and a Ph.D. from the University of Texas School of Public Health in Houston in 1977. He was a senior lecturer at the University of Nairobi, Department of Community Health until 1984. He joined UNICEF as Regional PHC Adviser based in Lusaka, Zambia, and became the Chief of Health Program, UNICEF Sudan.

Leo O. Ogba, Ph.D. is a senior lecturer in government and public administration at Imo State University, Nigeria. He was educated at the University of Ife and at the Norman Paterson School of International Affairs of Carleton University, Ottawa, Canada. His publications include a number of scholarly contributions to journals dealing with domestic security, intelligence, and public policy issues.

Tola Pearce, Ph.D. is a distinguished sociologist based at Ife, Nigeria. She has made extensive contributions to the study of health and family in the Third World.

R. Stock is a self-employed medical geographer with research interests in health and underdevelopment and Hausa traditional medicine. His address is 475 Bagot St., Kingston, Ontario, Canada.

P. A. Twumasi is professor of sociology at the University of Ghana. He is the editor for Africa of the influential journal *Social Science and Medicine*.

I. S. Ubot studied psychology at Loyola College in Balitmore, Maryland, USA where he obtained a B.A. degree in 1976 and an M.A. in Clinical Psychology in 1978. In 1982 he obtained a Ph.D. in psychology from Howard University. He also holds a Master of Public Health degree from Harvard University School of Public Health. Dr. Ubot has worked at the Institute for Social Research, University of Michigan, the Community College of Baltimore, Howard University, and the College of Medical Sciences, University of Calabar. Subsequently he worked at the University of Jos, Nigeria, where his research interests included the epidemiology and control of alcohol and drug abuse, health policy analysis, and social change and health.

For Polly Hill of the University of Cambridge
and Robin Law of the University of Stirling
for their contributions to African studies.

ACKNOWLEDGEMENTS

Toyin Falola would like to thank the staff of Clare Hall and the many libraries of the University of Cambridge who provided assistance when the manuscript was being edited for publication. Dennis Ityavyar would like to thank the staff of the library of the University of Toronto where he was able to gather materials for his chapters. Both of them acknowledge the financial support of Idowu Falola and the patience and interest of all the contributors to the volume. They also wish to acknowledge the encouragement received from the editors of *Social Science and Medicine* who gave them permission to reprint in a modified form two contributions previously published.

CONTENTS

Part I. INTRODUCTION

Part II. INDIGENOUS SYSTEMS AND COLONIAL HERITAGE

Part III: CONTEMPORARY CRISES AND CONTRADICTIONS

Part I: Introduction

1

THE CRISIS OF AFRICAN HEALTH CARE SERVICES

Toyin Falola

> Health of the mind and body is so fundamental to the good
> life that if we believe that men have any personal rights at
> all as human beings, then they have an absolute moral right
> to such a measure of good health as society and society
> alone is able to give them (Aristotle in *Politics*).

The World Health Organization (WHO) defines health as "a state
of complete physical, mental and social well-being and not merely
the absence of disease or infirmity." Some scholars have found this
definition lacking in operational appropriateness, and have
emphasized those conditions which promote "fulfilling and satisfy-
ing lives." Most definitions stress the quality of life of the
individual. No matter how health is defined, in Africa the state of
health care delivery is in crisis. Poor health care is part of the
overall crisis of underdevelopment in the continent. Unlike agriculture, it has received less attention from scholars. This book
attempts to examine this major aspect of African underdevelopment by focusing on the origin of the crisis as well as the major
aspects of the contemporary problems.

The volume is divided into three parts: Part I sets the
background, Part II concerns the introduction and consequences
of Western medicine, and Part III considers the major issues in
health care services.

From the Indigenous to the Western

The history of medicine in Africa has experienced many
overlapping phases, notably:

3

1. The era of ignorance, when little or nothing was known about the nature of diseases and how to cure them

2. The development of an indigenous system based on the understanding of diseases and the various ways to cure them

3. The spread of Arabic civilization, including its medical practices

4. The introduction of Western medical systems from the nineteenth century onwards;

5. The institutionalization of a curative system, especially after World War II

6. The search since the independence of African countries for the right approach to the health care crises, which includes (a) the retention of the colonial system; (b) the combination of both the curative and the preventive care; (c) "a free enterprise" approach in which individuals are abandoned to solve their problems in their own way; and (d) the recent concept of Primary Health Care which is gaining attention

Each phase involves specific features on the role of the individual, health workers, the state, the community, the understanding of the nature of illness and how to cure diseases, health awareness, the infrastructure for health care delivery, the economy of the society, and the share of resources that the state is willing to allocate to it.

In precolonial societies, the health care system stressed, among other things, the following features:

1. Diseases could come about through preternatural and supernatural causes (that is the machinations of enemies, the wrath of gods and witches)

2. Cures should deal with both the individual who was sick and the preternatural and supernatural agencies

3. Dealing with the preternatural and supernatural agencies involved sacrifices by the individual or the entire community

4. Health experts existed in every community, involving (a) elders in the households who relied on history and knowledge of medical problems in the household and (b) trained experts in different fields

4

5. The entire community involved itself in health care delivery by accepting the experts qualified to diagnose and prescribe, defining what constituted work and play, getting involved in environmental sanitation, planning and location of residential houses, markets, segregating the people who suffered from communicable diseases, integrating the just recovered back into the society and so forth

In this collection, chapters 2, 3, and 8 examine the main features of the indigenous system.

The introduction of Western (also called modern or orthodox) medicine to Africa was through the agency of the missionaries and the colonial government (Part I). The introduction was originally limited to the ports, and centers of administration and commerce. Expansion in medical facilities came after World War II when attempts were made to introduce reforms in order to forestall the emergence of aggressive nationalism. Part of the changes of the post-world war era was the provision of potable water, the concern with environmental hygiene and the expansion of hospitals as well as maternity, child welfare, and dispensary services. The colonial health delivery care system, however, was faced with an increasing volume of work, arising from new forms of poverty generated by colonialism.

Before its introduction into Africa, Western medicine had benefitted from the discovery of the germ theory, a growing knowledge of pathology, physiology and human anatomy, and technology brought about by the Industrial Revolution. Its mode of organization also benefitted from the concept of the state in the West and capitalist ideology. The neocolonial African states inherited the legacies of the colonial variant of Western medicine as well as both old and new diseases.

Both the manner of the introduction and the heritage of Western medicine brought new features and distortions to Africa. These included, among others, the following:

1. Emphasis on curative care which stressed the building of hospitals, dispensaries, and medical schools which followed the curricula of schools in the metropolises

2.   A curative approach which was very expensive for the patients involving their travelling to hospitals, paying bills, and buying drugs

3.   A diminished role for the community such that individuals no longer made contributions to the management of the health sector—the hospital with the physician in charge of the team work took over

4.   Difficult access to health care by the individual because of shortage of such things as hospitals, personnel, and drugs

5.   Inadequate coverage on a national basis—the preference was given to the cities, port towns, and seats of government

6.   An enormous growth in health problems, larger than could be solved by the strategies adopted. Though there were cases of improvement in some aspects, there were, at the same time, new problems generated by the penetration of Western capitalism

The Deepening Crisis

The crisis of underdevelopment in Africa has deepened in recent years. The World Bank report for 1983 indicated that the Gross National Product of thirty countries in the Third World was less than US $500 per person, nine countries had less than $1000, and three had between $1000 and $1500. Inflation had reached a double-digit rate in thirty-two countries.

In the face of falling prices, declining exports, and control by transnational companies, the economies of African countries exhibited retrogression rather than growth. In countries with minerals, the control over production lay with foreign firms. Because of heavy debts, the countries were under the firm grip of the International Monetary Fund with devastating consequences: devaluations, cuts in expenditures on health, education and social services, elimination of price controls, wage freezes, and so forth. Other problems have been discussed in recent literature on the continent.[1]

An editorial in the *Review of African Political Economy* (36:1986) catalogued the health impacts of this deepening crisis as follows:

1. High death rates reflected in extremely short lifespans. In 26 of 51 countries the average life expectancy at birth remained under 50 years. It was even under 40 years in 5 countries (Gambia, Guinea, Guinea Bissau, Somalia, and Sierra Leone)

2. Food shortage resulted in dearth of sustenance in 24 countries. Food production rose at less than half the population growth rate in the 1970s and actually declined by 15 percent between 1981 and 1983. Twenty percent of the population of sub-Saharan Africa depended on food imports and food aid. No fewer than 100 million people were thought to be malnourished. Mass starvation was reported in Eriteria, Ethiopia, Chad, Mozambique, and Sudan

3. With rising levels of deprivation the causes of death became non-specific and any acute infection was fatal. Death rates remained constant even when a disease such as smallpox was totally eradicated or full prevention had been achieved by total immunization such as against measles. When the burdens of poverty, crowding, malnutrition, and infection were great, the specific causes of death seemed to be interchangeable. Even the best health services appeared to make no impact when standards of living fell below subsistence levels

4. Africa had the highest birth rates in the world and the fastest growing population. Although most of the population was still rural, annual rates of urbanization ran over 4 percent. With more than 45 percent of the population under 15 years of age in almost all countries, the number of young and elderly dependents that had to be supported by the working population was extremely high; the dependency ratio (the combined population under fifteen and over sixty-four years as a percentage of the population between those ages) typically was over 90 percent in Africa, compared to 60 percent in the industrial market economies

The major diseases which attack and kill people (especially children) are fever, measles, pneumonia, whooping cough, gastro-enteritis, tuberculosis, malnutrition, anaemia, poliomyelitis, tetanus, and respiratory infections. Many studies have shown that several of these diseases are more prevalent among the lower socioeconomic groups. Poor living conditions and economic insecurity also have been associated with nervous breakdowns.[2]

Three hundred and fifty million people live in 'malarious' communities south of the Sahara.

The greatest threat today is against nutrition, the foundation of good health. Lack of adequate nutrition is related to food production which in Africa does not keep pace with population growth with the result that food prices have become prohibitive. Among the problems associated with nutrition are starvation, low protein consumption, malnutrition, and food-chemical pollution. These are accompanied by serious consequences: productivity is diminished; the learning process is inhibited; and the body resistance to diseases is destroyed.[3] Table 1 provides some health and development statistics in some of the developing countries of Africa for 1960 and 1982.

General data tend to obscure the magnitude of the problem in specific countries or even within areas of the same country. A few examples are provided here. In Angola in 1980, there were 797,688 reported cases of malaria, 390,507 cases of "other salmonella infections," 34,216 cases of bilharzioses, 54,126 cases of whooping cough, and 29,656 cases of measles. In the same year, the Republic of Benin reported 131,009 cases of malaria and 18,635 of measles. In Nigeria, a country with better economic resources, the top twenty killers listed in Table 2 were preventable. The 1981-1982 Nigeria Fertility Survey, a part of the World Fertility Survey, shows a crude death rate of 16 per thousand population, a crude birth rate of 48 per thousand population, an infant mortality rate of 85 per thousand live births, a maternal mortality rate of 15 per thousand live births, a childhood (1-4 year old) mortality rate of 60 per thousand live births, a mortality rate for people over five years old of 145 per thousand live births, and a life expectancy at birth of fifty-four years.[4]

Worse statistics have been described for South Africa, especially in the Bantustan communities of Transkei, Bophuthatswana, Venda, and Ciskei. The creation of these communities—the so-called independent homelands—involved stripping over eight million blacks of their citizenship by declaring them as aliens in South Africa and brought more suffering and repressions to the people. In the study of the Ciskei, Meredith Turshen pointed out that jobs were few, labor laws to protect workers' rights were nonexistent, food prices were high, overcrowding was the rule, and health conditions were very bad.[5] On health, Meredith supplied data on

8

Table 1

HEALTH AND DEVELOPMENT INDICATORS
IN SELECTED COUNTRIES 1960 AND 1982

Country	GNP per capita per year (US$) 1982	Average annual growth (%) 1960-1982	Debt Service as % of exports 1982	Life Expectancy at Birth 1960 M	1960 F	1982 M	1982 F	Infant Mortality (per 1000) 1960	1982
Chad	80	-2.8	0.4	33	36	42	45	210	161
Ethiopia	140	1.4	9.5	35	38	45	49	172	122
Zaire	190	-0.3	...	38	42	49	52	150	106
Tanzania	280	1.9	5.1	40	43	51	54	144	98
China	310	5.0	...	41	41	65	69	165	67
Kenya	390	2.8	20.3	45	48	55	59	112	77
Nigeria	860	3.3	9.5	37	40	48	52	190	109
Algeria	2350	3.2	24.6	46	48	55	59	165	111
South Africa	2670	4.9	...	51	55	60	65	92	55
France	11680	3.7	...	67	74	71	79	27	10
USA	13160	2.2	...	67	73	71	78	26	11

Source: ROAPE 36 (1986): 48.

9

Table 2

CAUSES OF MORBIDITY FROM DISEASE
IN NIGERIA, 1984-1986

Disease	1984		1985		1986	
	Number	Population per 10,000	Number	Population per 10,000	Number	Population per 10,000
Malaria	1,242,882	1,319.3	1,284,403	1,329.0	1,020,071	1,028.9
Dysentery (all types)	222,879	236.6	259,052	268.0	185,904	187.5
Measles	182,591	193.8	161,768	167.4	115,743	116.7
Pneumonia	101,455	107.7	120,285	124.5	82,312	83.0
Gonorrhoea	55,139	58.5	70,514	73.0	42,306	442.7
Whooping Cough	62,751	66.6	92,266	95.5	42,193	42.6
Schistosomiasias (all types)	36,710	39.0	31,788	32.9	26,975	27.2
Chicken Pox	65,932	70.0	76,226	78.9	21,387	21.6
Meningitis (both types)	1,302	1.4	1,425	1.5	17,168	17.3
Leprosy	8,800	9.3	8,293	8.6	14,659	14.8
Tuberculosis	10,677	11.3	14,934	15.5	14,071	14.2
Viral Influenza	5,941	6.3	18,156	18.8	9,991	10.1
Filariasis	12,746	13.5	16,586	17.2	9,247	9.3
Ophthalmianeonatorum	3,610	3.8	7,518	7.8	8,234	8.3
Food Poisoning	2,827	3.0	5,287	5.5	6,285	6.3
Infective - Hepatitis	5,316	5.6	7,647	7.9	3,766	3.8
Relapsing Fever	1,778	1.9	1,514	1.6	3,616	3.6
Trachoma	5,042	5.4	4,359	4.5	3,327	3.4
Tetanus	2,437	2.6	2,679	2.8	2,269	2.3
Onchocorciasis	5,046	5.4	7,317	7.6	1,994	2.0

Sources: Federal Republic of Nigeria, *Health Profile, 1986* (Lagos: Federal Ministry of Health, 1987).

infant mortality (50 percent), malnutrition (75 percent of urban and 80 percent of rural children), starvation (in 1983 Operation Hunger, a project of the South African Institute of Race Relations, had to feed 150,000 starving people a day), and the high rate of tuberculosis (2 percent of the adult population was affected). As in the other Bantustans, the conditions in Ciskei was aggravated by migrations in search of employment, inadequate arable land, and poor health services.

The causes of ill health in Africa have expanded also as a result of a general crisis in the economies of African countries. Chronic diseases have become common, and include malnutrition, stress, and AIDS. Stress was thought to be absent in Africa and an editorial in the Review of African Political Economy (ROAPE) offered an explanation for its occurrence as follows:

> Stress is a response to capitalist social relations; it is an expression of our reactions to the extraction of surplus from all social activity, not only from production at the workplace. Since the introduction of migratory labour systems this extension of extraction has been characteristic of capitalist development in Africa and has been denied by proponents of the economic theory of dualism for almost as long. Our failure to understand the nature of capital's strategy has led us to over emphasise processes like proletarianisation in our analysis of twentieth century developments in Africa and thus to overlook, until very recently, the exploitation of women and almost to miss the crisis of social reproduction.[6]

In 1986 Carol Barker and Meredith Turshen showed that AIDS had become a public health problem and that its reporting had been suppressed because of the need to protect the tourist industry and in response to Western attitudes which tended to blame the black race for its origin and spread. These two authors concluded that "health levels [were] deteriorating rapidly, malnutrition [was] spreading across the continent in the wake of the current drought, and Africans [were] more vulnerable to infections—now including AIDS—than ever before."[7]

The general health of Africans also is affected by the presence of counterfeit drugs. It is easy to sell fake drugs in Africa. The practice in most African countries is to walk to a drug store or to hawkers along the streets to buy drugs without any endorsed prescription by a doctor. The motive of drug sellers is profit. There are, of course, regulations on the sales of drugs classified as poison in many countries. Generally, these are expected to be sold to buyers with specific prescriptions from qualified medical personnel. The regulations are hardly enforced, however, because of the collusion between drug sellers and officials and the inability of health officials to monitor the sales of drugs.

Africa is a dumping ground for counterfeit drugs. These drugs are either imported from abroad or manufactured within Africa itself. Several techniques in faking have been discovered. There are cases of adulteration of pediatric syrups and capsules. In the case of capsules, empty capsule containers are imported and then filled with all sorts of powders (such as baby food formula and dusting powder) and sold as drugs. Expired drugs generally are sold, either with the expiry date still on them or, more usually, by repackaging and the addition of new expiry dates. Another form of pharmaceutical fraud is to invent names that are close to an established drug or trademark name. For example, Septrin syrup is imitated in many places under names such as New Septrin, Septrim, Septrink, Setrin, and Semptrin. The new packages also imitate the original. Cases of repacking are too common: for instance a drug in 200mg container can be repacked into small containers with misleading labels.

Self medication and noncompliance with medical instructions also are widespread. The reasons are many: ignorance; the high cost of consulting a doctor; lack of access to medical facilities; influence of people who have successfully used a drug and who recommend it to others; the time lost in hospitals, especially by those who have no connections with the staff; very easy access to drug stores and hawkers; and reliance on "cure all" capsules.

Impostors also are many. Hospital orderlies, cleaners, and nurses pose as competent doctors. There are instances of clinics being operated by quacks. The activities of these fake personnel flourish because of widespread ignorance on the part of the patients, the elitism that characterizes the structure of health care services, the cheapness of services offered by quacks, and the

12

problems of access to genuine personnel. The dearth of personnel is too well known to elaborate upon here. It is certain that the continent cannot attain the World Health Organization (WHO) recommendation of a ratio of one doctor per 10,000 people by the year 2000. Nurses, radiologists, radiographers, and pharmacists are all in short supply.

Another major threat to health stems from the dumping of toxic waste containing highly poisonous radioactive materials. The danger posed to both humans and plants by radioactive wastes is enormous because their radiation damages plant and animal tissue. Gamma rays, for instance, alter the nature of some body cells and cause cancer.[8] A 1988 report by the International Atomic Energy Agency (IAEA) based in Vienna, Austria shows clearly that the problem of disposal and storage of 0.5 million tons of radioactive waste is yet to be solved. Thirty-three countries have generated such poisonous wastes since the 1960s. But as the IAEA reports, no country has built safe storage facilities. With 106 nuclear reactors, the U.S. has the largest amount of radioactive waste. It is followed by the USSR. There is a total of fifteen nuclear waste reprocessing plants in the world, three each in France, the U.S., and India, two in Britain and one each in Japan, China, Italy, and Germany. Though these countries have identified safe sites, only the underground repository being built by Germany will be ready in 1999. The U.S. has chosen a site in Nevada but this will not become functional until the next century. The ideal storage for poisonous wastes consists of a very deep excavation in an area where the rocks are stable, impermeable, and not prone to earthquake. Such underground excavations are lined and the wastes, in very thick steel containers, are buried permanently.

Deep burial is an expensive undertaking and it attracts litigation by people in areas chosen as sites so that it is cheaper for waste producers to dump wastes in Africa in collusion with useless and corrupt members of the ruling class. Under such circumstances, producers need not worry about litigation, damage to the environment and proper procedures for disposal. As some recent cases have indicated, producers simply dump the wastes on beaches. Different methods have been used in this dangerous toxic waste traffic. One involved the negotiations with the governments of certain countries. Under a tight grip of Western control and financial expediency, these countries see nothing wrong in exchanging money for death and disease.

Some of the countries which engaged in deals on toxic waste are now known. *La Lettre du Continent*, a France-based confidential newsletter, reported the case of Gabon and the Central Africa Republic (CAR) in its June 1988 edition. In 1987, Gabon established a plan for a treatment plant for toxic waste. This plant, called The Nuclear Waste Disposal Centre would be located in Panga, fifteen miles north of Mayumba in the southern part of the country. It would have a capacity to store 120,000 tons of low and medium radioactive waste a year. It is expected that 60,000 tons would be deposited in 1990, and 90,000 in 1991. In anticipation of more waste, the plant's capacity could be extended to 240,000 tons per annum. The choice of Panga was not without its reasons among which were (a) the availability of independent port facilities, (b) unlimited land availability, (c) excellent living conditions, (d) ideal geology and hydro-geological system, (e) good logistical support and telecommunication system, and (f) accessibility to the sources of waste—Panga can be reached from Europe and the United States. The reason announced in the country was that the center would publicly contribute to economic development and scientific knowledge. The Gabonese government announced that the center would develop research and educational facilities for Gabon and other African countries. To achieve these advertised goals, the government decided to establish the Societe Gabonaise d'Etudes Nucleaires to organize the new facilities and finance Le Centre International of Panga.

In the case of CAR a contract was signed in 1985 by "highly placed citizens" and some European businessmen to buy toxic waste (both industrial and pharmaceutical) in Bakouma region. This would be done at the rate of $40 per ton. The first shipment of 70,000 tons was made in 1986; the contents were described as agricultural fertilizers. Since 1986, an annual shipment of between 60,000 and 70,000 tons has been reported.

Other countries that have imported waste (chemical or toxic) include Benin, Congo, Equatorial Guinea, Morocco, Guinea, Djibouti, Guinea Bissau, Nigeria, Senegal, Zimbabwe, Sierra Leone, and South Africa. Some of these countries were involved in the negotiations for these wastes while some received them without the knowledge of their governments. The case of Nigeria is

14

particularly noteworthy.[9] In May of 1988, when the Nigerian head of state was organizing a declaration by the Organization of African Unity (OAU) against toxic dumping, he did not realize that an Italian company had already dumped waste at Koko, a small port in Bendel state. The number of cases of illegal dumping are not known, but there are companies that specialize in dumping activities. These companies exploit their knowledge of the movements on high seas, the ignorance of host governments, the corruption of officials, smuggling, and the "grey area of international legislation" to organize their business. Officials of the International Register of Potentially Toxic Chemicals believe that Africa has been receiving large shipments of toxic waste since the 1970s. The particulars of the companies involved in the transactions are either unknown or dubious. Even when these companies are known, they cannot be punished by their home governments because they have not broken local rules.

The OAU declared in May 1988 that members would refrain from entering into agreements with any industrialized country, transnational corporation, private company or interest groups on the dumping of nuclear and hazardous wastes on African territories. At the regional level the 1988 meeting of the ECOWAS Authority (made up of heads of states) also passed resolutions on waste dumping.[10] In spite of these two collective decisions, some countries were unwilling to terminate their contracts because of the money they would lose. Equatorial Guinea, Guinea Bissau, Benin, Congo, and Gabon are among these "stubborn" countries. Without any regional, continental, or international legislation to protect the continent, individual countries may have to decide on punitive actions against waste dealers. The continent should insist that those who produce the waste should keep it in their countries.

Chapter 10 raises the issue of inequality in the access to health. As far back as 1946, WHO put into its constitution the necessity of equal access: "the enjoyment of the highest attainable standard of health is one of the fundamental rights of every human being without distinction of race, religion, political belief, economic or social conditions." But as Tola Pearce says in this chapter, the problem of inequality is a big one. Other data support the conclusions reached by Pearce. There is a high degree of inadequacy in health care facilities, both in manpower and physical

15

facilities, with the result that thousands of people simply do not have access to modern medical facilities. A number of studies have shown that one factor for the massive rural-urban migrations is the need to have access to health facilities. Recent studies show that such access is becoming difficult. Not all African countries have medical schools to train personnel. Where the schools exist, the products are not enough. In many countries less than 30 percent of the population enjoy access to health care facilities. Access is affected by such factors as availability of facilities, cost of care, location of facilities, cost of transportation, and availability of alternate traditional systems. In most countries, rural areas suffer most from these inadequacies. Most figures on personnel and budgets fail to reveal that these are concentrated in the cities.

Inequality exists in both rural and urban areas. Facilities in the villages, where they exist, are poorly utilized because such places are poorly managed (that is, drugs are scarce, staff are inadequate, and provision for emergency services is lacking).[11] Yet the bulk of the African population (about 75 percent) live in rural areas. Several studies have shown that these villages are not served by medical facilities.[12] The problems of the rural areas are compounded by a poor transportation system. In the cities, urban hospitals fulfill their referral functions inadequately. The reason is that they usually serve the interests of city-dwellers by concentrating on the treatment of both minor and major cases. Urban hospitals are too few for the population they serve with the result that at the out-patient departments there always is overcrowding, a scarcity of drugs, poor attention to patients, overworking of staff, and incivility by hospital staff. While the poor have to cope with these problems, the better-off can patronize private clinics which have become better developed.

National budgetary allocations to the health sector remain unsatisfactory. Financial allocations are generally small—below 2 percent of the total annual budgets in many countries. Generally they are unstable, fluctuating from year to year. The bulk of financial allocations to health usually goes to curative services. Primitive accumulation by the ruling class has penetrated the health sector: contracts are inflated, drugs are expensive, and money meant for health is diverted into private pockets. Political instability, wars and other forms of violence also have taken their toll on health finances. The impact of violence forms the subject

16

of attention in chapter 9. Violence has led to the destruction of health care infrastructures, and the diversion of personnel to the emergency treatment of victims of violence. Where progress has been recorded in health policy, as in the case of Mozambique, it has been retarded by war and aid donors who disrupt central planning.

Underdevelopment has pushed the continent into the degrading status of a beggar for aid in forms of drugs, food, personnel, and technology. Medical aid agencies dominated by non-governmental organizations (NGOs) are now sought. These donors include UNICEF, WHO, FAO, the World Bank, the EC, USAID, and hundreds of others. These organizations are diverse in their activities and primary intention. There are "those who want to.act against injustice and inequality and those who have recourse to aid in order to preserve the present international economic order on which the North's growth is based."[13] The diversity is reflected in the projects they sponsor, ranging from population control projects, distribution of drugs, and construction of health centers to the supply of free food.

The impact of aid seems to have been ignored by the desperate African countries in search of quick remedies and forget that pain killers have side effects. Annie Tae'baud poses an excellent question on the impact of aid.

> How can a country construct a coherent health policy on the basis of a national strategy, as WHO recommends, when international experts are placed in ministries, when medical volunteers of more than fifty nationalities are working individually or in organized missions and when the workers of multiple micro-projects developed by hundreds of NGOs of different nationalities and different professional, political, and ideological perspectives are all operating in one and the same country.[14]

The answer is very obvious.

> Even though a cost-benefit analysis is impossible, one wonders what part of this change is due to inter-national aid. Enduring improvements in health status

depend essentially on the internal social dynamics of a country and the political choices it has made, including its relations with the world economic system of which international aid is a part.[15]

After noting that China has improved its health status, he concluded that

the problem posed by international aid and its perverse effects is situated at a much more fundamental level: aid is an integral part of the relations of domination between the countries of the North and the countries of the South. The real political move is not to suppress aid for its own sake but to transform the economic, social, and political relations, not only between industrialized countries and the third world, but within each society, North and South. The struggle against health inequalities is on the social agenda of transformation necessary in all societies.[16]

A big problem often ignored in the literature is the violation of human rights. Detention without trial is so common in the African continent. Detainees experience psychological and physical sickness. Denial of democratic rights also affects health. People are brutally attacked when they fight for their rights, and their lives are affected when they are prevented from fighting for their rights of working towards the enhancement of their quality of life. Health cannot be separated from socio-political conditions. The conclusion by Meredith in the case of Ciskei applies to the continent.

The provision of good health services does not depend so much on the skill of health workers as on prevailing economic, social, and political conditions. For example, South African pediatricians may have developed an expertise in the understanding and treatment of malnutrition and its complications, but medical expertise does not change the system that gives rise to malnutrition nor the environment to which treated children return, an environment in which half the children die before their fifth birthday. Malnutrition, in

18

this context, is a direct result of the government's policies, which perpetuate the apartheid system and promote the poor health conditions and human rights violations.[17]

To sum up the problems of the health system in Africa include the following:

1. The capitalist orientation of the health care delivery system
2. Violation of human rights
3. Inadequate population coverage by the medical services
4. Rural-urban imbalance in the provision of medical facilities
5. Inadequate use of existing facilities
6. Underdevelopment of traditional health care system
7. Manpower shortage
8. Lack of proper coordination of the different components of the health program
9. The prevalence of preventable diseases
10. Self-medication, dumping of fake drugs, and toxic wastes
11. The general socioeconomic underdevelopment of the continent

Attempts at Solution

The curative approach has been the main focus of attention in health care policies since World War II. The bulk of the money spent, the arguments on strategy, as well as the plans adopted all have emphasized cure, rather than prevention. Two strategies have dominated attention, (a) the provision of medical education and medical personnel and (b) the development of medical infrastructures and technology. The success of these two strategies always has been measured in terms of health and related indicators such as data on life expectancy and the number of doctors per one thousand population.

The curative approach has had several problems, including (a) the inability to accept the fact that good health is associated with good food, hygienic environment, and the provisions of basic amenities such as clean water; (b) modern medical facilities while

19

they have made it possible and easier to cure several diseases, in Africa, they have increased the cost of health care services beyond what the majority of the population can afford. Policy based on spending the bulk of the budget on medical technology ends up catering for an affluent few; and (c) lessons from the indigenous system have been ignored. Arising from the failure of the preventive approach, the criticisms of scholars, complaints by millions of people on their state of health, and contributions by the World Health Organization, attention has shifted in recent time to epidemiological issues, based on the concern for prevention, rather than cure.

As chapter 11 indicates, there are a few cases of non-capitalist national health policies. Though they have had their problems, the non-capitalist approach offers another model. The case of Mozambique has been documented, and but for the protracted struggle for independence and development, struggles which involve war, perhaps better progress would have been recorded. Health received priority attention after Mozambique's independence. The country nationalized health care in 1975 and launched a national program on sanitation in the following year. In 1977, it established a National Drug Formulary. In the same year, the health policy of the nation was stated clearly. It gave every individual the responsibility of a sanitary agent as well as the power "to arm and organize people to defend themselves and their health." The policy banned private medicine which was regarded as "a means of exploitation which used diseases to accumulate wealth." The policy also emphasized preventive medicine. "The development of preventive medicine [was] the principal priority for the Ministry of Health. It correspond[ed] to the fundamental needs and capacity of the country. In this context, [the country was to] continue to develop actions aimed at the sanitary and nutritional education of the people and the improvement of environmental sanitation."[18] Though the overall goal of health for all is yet to be realized, this policy showed an understanding of the problems, especially among the people.[19]

By the end of the 1980s, the advertised objectives of health services in so many countries are aimed at providing protective, promotional, restorative, and rehabilitative services. In some countries with so-called comprehensive health care the program is supposed to operate at three levels: (a) tertiary health care which

20

is to concentrate in teaching and specialist hospitals and schools and undertake research into aspects of health and the training of personnel for the other two levels; (b) secondary health care to provide referral services and assist in specialized cases; and (c) primary health care to focus on services provided by health centers, clinics, and out-patient departments of hospitals in both rural and urban centers.

The most prominent of this three-tiered approach is the primary health care (PHC) strategy. PHC was not the invention of an African country. Rather, it arose as part of a universal concern for the plight of the poor. Its architect was WHO and it originated in the Declaration of Alma-Ata at a conference in 1978.[20] The basis to achieve "health for all by the year 2000" through PHC was as follows:

1. Mass literacy and education of the people on health problems in their areas and simple ways to prevent and control them

2. Promotion of food supply and proper nutrition

3. Giving adequate supply of safe water and basic sanitation

4. Maternal and child health care, including family planning. In this context, family planning refers to services offered to couples to educate them about family life and to encourage them to achieve their wishes with regard to (a) preventing unwanted pregnancies, (b) securing desired pregnancies, (c) spacing pregnancies, and (d) limiting the size of the family's health and socioeconomic status. The methods prescribed should be compatible with their culture and religious beliefs

5. Immunization of people against the major infectious diseases

6. Prevention and control of locally endemic and epidemic diseases

7. Giving of appropriate treatment to common diseases and injuries

8. Provision of essential drugs and supplies

From the above objectives, PHC recognizes the role of prevention, basic human needs, better diet, inter-sectoral and community participation, education, and self-reliance. The objectives of the

21

PHC stress social justice, equity, and socially and economically productive lives.

Of all the major aspects of departure between the curative approach and the PHC strategy, community participation is the most important. As the Alma-Ata Declaration put it, it is "the process by which individuals and families assume responsibility for their own health and welfare for those of the community and develop the capacity to contribute to them and the community's development." For this participation to be meaningful, it should involve everybody irrespective of the level of education, sex, race, religion, and color. Community participation is important mainly because it gives the people the power to participate and even challenge the decisions taken on its behalf. It is however, a concession that would be granted most reluctantly, if at all.

The World Health Organization wisely insisted that the performance of PHC should be evaluated and monitored in all countries.[21] WHO took steps to formulate guidelines. Evaluation and monitoring would make it possible to know if gains had been made and to correct lapses. Part of the monitoring should include the production of maps for different communities so as to know the locations of villages and towns; the number of houses; the census and numbering of households and its members; the monitoring of children's growth; the evaluation of the performance of personnel; and the adequacy of facilities.

The attitude to PHC varied from one country to the other. A few countries actually announced PHC as their official health policy. Nigeria, for instance, integrated it into its development, with the following objectives:

1.   To initiate the provision of adequate and effective health facilities and care for the entire population

2.   To correct the imbalances in the location and distribution of health institutions

3.   To correct the imbalance between preventive and curative medicine

4.   To provide the infrastructure for all preventive health programs such as the control of communicable diseases, family health, environmental health, nutrition, and school health

5.   To establish a health care system best adapted to the level of health technology and financial resources of the country[22]

These objectives have remained at the level of rhetoric.

In Mozambique emphasis has been put on central planning of which PHC is a part, being adopted in 1978. Setbacks in the execution of PHC have been apparent. For example, village health workers have abandoned their work, the democratization of the hospitals has been put into second place with priority given to stronger management so that in many areas the results of health care in terms of better health are less than tangible. Progress has been recorded in such matters as the attempt to manufacture drugs locally, the building of thousands of latrines in cities and villages, the provision of PHC centers (there were 1,371,443 in 1984), the increase in the number of health workers in the provinces, and the training of new paramedical workers. Some of these belonged to the Cadre d'Agentes Polivalentes Elementares (APE)—the equivalent of barefoot doctors. The expectations of the APE have not been met mainly because of the war of liberation which destroyed many villages.[23] The principles underlying PHC should not be abandoned even though PHC and other aspects of health are experiencing difficulties in Mozambique, especially from pressure to adapt to donor policy preferences, and from pressures to neglect sectors which lack donor-appeal for lack of sovereign funds, as well as economic pressure, war, and the policy on health. Cliff, Kanji, and Muller concluded that

> it has been demonstrated that the health care system introduced by Frelimo can, given a fair chance, serve people's need. It offers a way of using scarce resources fairly and effectively—and the scarcer they are the more important it is that they be used in the most effective manner possible. The only real alternative is to abandon the people to the Curandeiro and the Farmacia and go back to the bad old days of second-rate medicine for profit for those who can afford it and nothing for the vast majority.[24]

Schoept has provided a reliable report on Zaire. He pointed to the class and urban bias of health services: the government hospital at Kinshasa consumed over half of the national health budget and the bourgeoisie has access to routine biomedical care. Interest groups, political elite, doctors, and so forth pay little attention to the objectives of PHC. "Under these circumstances," he concluded, "a PHC programme is likely to serve the rural (or urban) poor only in exceptional circumstances. More probably, its resources will be used in the main as capital to promote office-holders and local elites into the ranks of the state bourgeoisie."[25] In most other countries, the strategy has been to choose one or two aspects of PHC and ignore the rest. When there is assistance from foreign agencies, immunization of children is carried out such as UNICEF's Expanded Immunization Programme.

The implementation of PHC has been hampered by many factors which include, among others, the following:

1.   Inadequate political commitment to the concept. While some governments pay lip service to free and comprehensive services, some simply regard the health sector as a burden. Many countries have no positive progress to report. In countries with reports, the ruling class concentrates on aspects where money can be made by them as part of their own strategy of enrichment and consolidation. Governments also have redefined PHC to suit their own purposes

2.   Inadequate finance. Generally, financial allocation to health falls below the 5% of total budget as recommended by WHO. The emphasis is still on asking patients to pay with excep-tions granted to the children and, in a few cases, to the needy such as the disabled and the chronically ill (cancer and mental illness)

3.   Failure to follow the multisectoral approach suggested by PHC. If PHC is not planned together with other sectors such as agriculture and housing, there can be no meaningful development

4.   Lack of training of personnel to work in the rural areas

5.   Inadequate infrastructure in terms of building and appropriate tools

6.   Management problems in relation to the use of resources and collection of data

7.   Emphasis on curative health. The political leadership stands to benefit from this by purchasing drugs from abroad and building hospitals, both of which involve contracts and the massive corruption that accompanies them. Contracts also encourage the penetration and consolidation of multinational companies such as drug suppliers, builders and advisers on policy matters. Those who benefit from these contacts continue to measure improved health

by the indices of increase in hospitals, doctors, and equipment. This is a deliberate propaganda to cover their real intentions

8. Constraints posed by the vested interests of curative-oriented physicians, drug sellers, and officials. Govan Sterky has shown that physicians tend to resist approaches that diminish medicine as the major component of health policy[26]

On the whole, the impact of PHC is yet to be felt, especially on correcting the ills of the health system. PHC has to use more people at the grassroots and understand the common diseases in every community so as to know the best strategy to adopt. PHC must be organized not purely as a health system but as a combination of health and community development plan which would solve the problems of basic human needs. Most efforts in Africa today fail to suggest an intent to achieve the minimum requirements of PHC. Rather, policies are taken either in response to demands (stifling conditionalities) of creditors, or of peripheral capitalist development. Among the recent health policies are the emphasis on propaganda to reduce population growth through family planning, payment in hospitals for consultation and drugs encouragement of private clinics, and cuts in expenditure. Added to these is the migration of skilled personnel from the continent.

There has been an effort calling for a re-definition of PHC through "selective health strategies" which involve "a temporary alternative to PHC for all . . . deciding only to provide limited (and normally only preventive health care) interventions, rather than to provide an integrated system of care." The emphasis of the selective approach would be to prevent or treat diseases which cause death. The argument of the proponents of the selective approach was based on cost and coercion; that PHC was too expensive and called for too much intervention by government to the extent that individual freedom might be curtailed.[27] The selective approach has been justifiably criticized by WHO and condemned by scholars who regarded it as an approach that would further lead to the underdevelopment of health services in Africa.[28]

The Need for a Revolution

There is an urgent need for a revolution in health services in Africa which would jettison the negative aspects of Western medicine and emphasize preventive services. It has become clear that curative approach is expensive and yields little result. The diseases that kill more than 50 percent of the African population (malaria, measles, tetanus, tuberculosis, meningitis, gastroenteritis, cholera, and dysentery) can be attacked best by a preventive approach. Public and environmental health deserves more attention than it has received. According to WHO, public health

> is the science and art of preventing diseases, prolonging life, and promoting mental and physical health and efficiency through organised community efforts for the sanitation of the environment, the control of infections, the education of the individual in personal hygiene, the organization of medical and nursing services for the early diagnosis and preventive treatment of disease, and the development of social machinery to ensure to everybody a standard of living adequate for the maintenance of health so organizing these benefits as to enable every citizen to realise his birth-right of health and longevity.[29]

WHO suggests an environmental health scheme to solve several of the common diseases. Proper implementation of the scheme would involve the provision of good water supply, good methods of waste disposal, pest and vector control, personal and public hygiene, solid wastes management, air pollution, and noise control. The control of dangerous chemicals and toxic wastes has to be part of any major scheme on environmental health. Health education should be embarked upon at the same time. The purpose is to imbibe the knowledge of how to solve common health problems and participate in community programs.

African countries must take control over drug production so as to reduce cost and guarantee quality. The purchase of drugs is one of the ways of private accumulation of wealth through the state. It enables the transfer of wealth to the West and prevents the building of a viable pharmaceutical industry. Yet the resources for drugs are abundant. Of the $83.5 billion which the United Nations estimated to be the total world production of pharmaceuticals in 1980, Africa accounted for only 0.6 percent but consumed 2.3 percent, an amount equivalent to 400 percent of its own production.[30] The huge bill for drug purchases rather than improving the health of Africans has fostered the growth of foreign pharmaceutical companies which are noted for the over-invoicing of their products and wasteful expenditure on advertisements. The activities of these companies must be curtailed by reducing the number of competing products, bulk purchase of essential drugs, and the creation of indigenous pharmaceutical industries.

There is no escape from providing more infrastructure and personnel. The provision of both of these should be cost-effective and take care of the people in both rural and urban areas. There is an urgent need for a creative use of traditional healers. For this is needed a careful inventory of the healers and their practices, a scientific assessment of traditional medical knowledge to enhance their quality, and an understanding of the different perspectives on the etiology of disease causation. Chapters 3 and 8 have tried to show that there are values in the indigenous system and that traditional practitioners of all sorts can be employed. These include bone setters, herbalists, spiritualists, naturalists, circumcisors, midwives, as well as snake and scorpion bite specialists.

There are compelling reasons why traditional medical systems have to be recognized; many aspects of them are relevant to contemporary society. Chapters 3 and 8 stress that the indigenous systems concentrate on prevention and community participation in the overall health care delivery system. Moreover, some people (those in the villages and the urban poor) patronize traditional healers. This patronage has to do with cultural beliefs and attitudes which still accord importance and respect to such healers.[31] These beliefs rest partly on the understanding of diseases which attribute their causes to supernatural powers.[32] Even when people go to hospitals, they at the same time use traditional medicine as a complement. The efficacy of many of the traditional drugs have been confirmed, even in the difficult cases of psychiatric disorder and bone injury, not to mention common diseases such as malaria, fever, and headache. The contributions of traditional systems have been recognized also in such complicated cases as mental illness.[33]

The attempt to use traditional healers and their medicine will of course generate problems. Western-trained doctors criticize traditional doctors and are not likely to accept them. There are also problems about the approach to be adopted in making use of traditional healers. Some people have suggested incorporation or integration. The main problem in any approach will lie with the distribution of power. As chapter 3 points out, traditional healers had power during the precolonial era. The introduction of Western medicine gradually robbed them of their power and the access to decision-making. This was a great loss which made them confine their activities to the realm of private practice. Perhaps it was part of the strategy of regaining control of the private sphere that has pushed traditional healers to place primary emphasis on their supernatural power, sometimes at the expense of the tangible scientific components of their healing activities. As long as traditional healers play a secondary role they will continue to seek means of distorting their profession in the quest for power and control over the patients who patronize them. At the end of the 1980s, not many people were receiving training as traditional medical practitioners, the conclusion having been reached that ethno-medical practitioners could not be turned out in adequate numbers to make them viable additions to the health care delivery system.[34] In the rural areas, the recruitment of new people is affected by migration, the impacts of Christianity and Islam which condemn traditional medicine, and low financial remunerations to practitioners. The introduction of Western education has weakened the practice of apprenticeship; the younger generation prefer to go to schools.

In addition to the traditional healers, the use of barefoot doctors also has been suggested. It is common knowledge that the ailments which affect most people do not require the services of doctors with long training. China has solved the dearth of personnel by using barefoot doctors at less financial cost.[35] The practice has encouraged the democratization of health delivery systems. China's experience can be improved upon in the areas of uniformity of training, supervisions, and control of personnel. The army of the unemployed school graduates in Africa could be mobilized and trained to perform the functions of barefoot doctors. These cheap but competent personnel could form a very strong core of rural healers. Similar to traditional doctors of old, they would live in the communities. The continent cannot wait for good health until adequate orthodox doctors have been trained. Citizens should be mobilized in a vigorous campaign for environmental work to exterminate flies and protect sources of drinking water.

Finally, for a viable program on health to produce desired results, there must be an overall transformation of society. It is unlikely that the health sector can develop when the agricultural sector does not, when politics remains unstable, and when the transport system is poor. There can be no solution to the problems of health in Africa unless the linkage between poverty and health is recognized. Programs should not just limit themselves to increasing the number of facilities and personnel but should be concerned with raising the general standard of living. Since most diseases have been associated with poor living conditions, governments must provide the basic necessities of life. The poor have to be liberated. Today, the difficulty of living and rising cost of living brings more diseases to the poor. The health of the people of Africa will continue to be affected by economic and political conditions and by the overall popular resistance for change, reforms, and radical transformation. The struggle for improved health entails the struggle for freedom, the transformation of the continent, and the liquidation of the imperialist domination of the health sector in Africa.

NOTES

1. See for instance Bade Onimode, *A Political Economy of the African Crisis* (London: Zed, 1988).
2. Review of African Political Economy (ROAPE), 36 (September 1986): pp. 3-4.
3. L. Timberlate, *Africa in Crisis: The Causes, the Cures of Environmental Bankruptcy* (London: Earthscan, 1985), p. 50.
4. D. A. Jaiyeola, *Hints on the Principles of Psychiatry and Psychiatric Nursing Practice* (Ile-Ife: Obafemi Awolowo University Press, 1987).
5. M. Turshen, "Health and Human Rights in a South African Bantustan," *Social Science and Medicine* 22/9 (1986): 887-92.
6. ROAPE, 36, p. 4.
7. Ibid., p. 54.
8. For a recent study on the impact of toxic wastes, see Michael R. Edelstein, *Contaminated Communities: The Social and Psychological Impacts of Residential Toxic Exposure* (Boulder: Westview Press, 1988).
9. See the newspaper West Africa, 20 June 1988.
10. These are that (a) the sixteen-member organization agreed to enact laws in their respective countries making it a criminal offence to dump toxic waste on their territories; (b) the organization resolved to tighten controls on exporters of the toxic rubbish who are hampered in their home countries by tight environmental legislations; and (c) the organization agreed to set up a monitoring system, called "dump watch" under which members would alert each other of attempts to dump waste in their dominions.
11. See *Nigerian National Development Plan, 1981-1985*; A. I. Odebiyi and T. O. Pearce, "Health Care Development Strategy and Crisis: The Nigerian Case," *Nigerian Journal of Economic and Social Studies* 22/2 (1980): 17-37; and R. L.

Morrill and R. J. Earickson, "Problems in Modelling Interaction: The Case of Hospital Care," in *Behavioural Problems in Geography: A Symposium*, ed. K. Cox and R. G. Golledge (Evaston, Illinois: Northwestern University, 1969).

12. See P. A. Twumasi, *Medical Systems in Ghana* (Accra: Ghana Publishing Co., 1975) and O. Adejuyigbe, *The Location of the Rural Basic Health Facilities in Ife-Ijesha Area of South Western Nigeria* (Ile-Ife: University of Ife, 1977), Introduction.

13. J. Bryant, *Health and the Developing World* (Ithaca: Cornell University Press, 1967); F. Mburu, "Phetoric-Implementation Gap In Health Policy and Health Service Delivery For A Rural Population In A Developing Country," *Social Science and Medicine* 13A/5 (1972): 577-83.

14. ROAPE, 36, p. 45.

15. Ibid., p. 46.

16. Ibid., p. 48.

17. Ibid., p. 49.

18. Turshen, "Health and Human Rights," p. 891.

19. Julie Cliff, Najimi Kanji, and Mike Muller, "Mozambique Health Holding the Line" in ROAPE, 36, pp. 3-23.

20. Declaration of Alma-Ata, *Primary Health Care, Report of the International Conference on Primary Health Care, Alma-Ata, USSR, 6-12 September* (Geneva: WHO, 1978). The Conference was jointly sponsored by WHO and UNICEF.

21. Ibid.

22. Nigeria, *Third National Development Plan*, 1980-85.

23. Cliff, Kanji, and Muller, "Mozambique," p. 7.

24. Ibid., p. 22.

25. B. G. Schocpt, "Primary Health Care In Zaire," ROAPE, 36, p. 58.

26. Govan Sterky, "Towards another Development in Health," *Development Dialogue* 1 (1978): 1.

27. ROAPE, 36, pp. 78-84.

28. World Health Organization, *Technical Report Series No. 47* (Geneva: WHO, 1952) and *Afro Technical Series No. 5* (Brazaville: WHO, 1973).

29. World Health Organization, *Measurement in Health Promotion and Protection* (Geneva: WHO, 1987), pp. 35-36.

30. United Nations Centre on Transnational Corporations, *The Pharmaceutical Industry of Developing Countries* (New York: United Nations, 1984): 3-4.

31. See A. I. Odebiyi, "Socio-Cultural Factors Affecting Health Care Delivery in Nigeria," *Tropical Medicine and Hygiene* 80 (1980): 240-54; G. J. Ebrahim, *Care of the New Born in Developing Countries* (London: Macmillan, 1979); C. M. U. Maclean, *Social and Community Medicine for Students* (London: Heinemann, 1971); and A. H. Leighton, T. A. Lambo, C. C. Hughes, D. C. Leighton, J. M. Murphy and H. B. Macklin, *Psychiatric Disorders Among the Yoruba* (New York: Cornell University Press, 1963).

32. O. A. Erinosho and N. W. Bell (eds.), *Mental Health in Africa* (Ibadan: Ibadan University Press, 1982); A. Chambwe, "Psychological and Psychiatric Services in Zimbabwe," *Bulletin of the British Psychological Society* 35 (July 1982); A. Kiev (ed.), *Magic, Faith and Healing* (New York: Free Press, 1964); U. Maclean, *Magical Medicine: A Nigerian Case Study* (Middlesex: Penguin, 1971); P. A. Twumasi, "The Parsonian Sick Role Formulation and Illness Behaviour in Ghana," *Ghana Social Science Journal* 3/2 (Nov. 1976): 26-35; and S. Feirman, "Struggles for Control: The Social Roots of Health and Healing in Modern Africa," *African Studies Review* 28 (1985): 33-147.

33. Leighton, Lambo, et al., *Psychiatric Disorder*; T. Harding, "Psychosis in a Rural West African Community," *Social Psychiatry* 8 (1973); and R. O. A. Makanjuola, "Traditional and Religious Medicine: A Valid Alternative to Modern Medicine?" Mimeo.

34. C. Anyinam, "Traditional Medical Practice in Contemporary Ghana: A Dying or Growing 'Profession'?" *Canadian Journal of African Studies* 21/3 (1987): 315-36. See also G. M. Foster, "Anthropological Research and Perspectives on Health Problems in Developing Countries," *Social Sciences and Medicine* 18 (1984): 847-54.

35. V. W. Sidel, "Barefoot Doctors of the People's Republic of China," *New England Journal of Medicine* (1972): 1292-1300, and M. Rosenthal and J. R. Greines, "The Barefoot Doctors of China: From Political Creation to Professionalization," *Human Organization* 41/4 (1982).

Part II: Indigenous Systems and Colonial Heritage

2

HEALTH IN PRECOLONIAL AFRICA

Dennis A. Ityavyar

Before A.D. 1800, European powers had colonized no part of the African continent. The various peoples in the continent were organized into chiefdoms, empires, kingdoms, and autonomous states. For instance in the area south of the Sahara, there existed several great empires and kingdoms such as Ethiopia, Kanem-Borno, Asante, Mali, Songhai, and Oyo. Further south in the present central and southern African regions there were the Luba-Luna states, Buganda, Bunyoro, Rwanda, the Kongo, the Zulu and the Mwenemutapa empires. Beside the great empires and kingdoms there were several autonomous states in all parts of Africa such as the Igbo, Tiv, Sotho, and Nguni. The latter were non-centralized states.

As is true of all human societies, the development of precapitalist Africa was influenced by four closely "intertwined areas of human activity: the political, the socio-economic, the cultural, and the medical."[1] All these activities can be summarized into what we have chosen to call the precapitalist African mode of production. The economy within this mode was buoyant, with the family as the basic and simplest unit of production. The family provided for the protection and rights of its members. Families with a common descent formed a clan. A cluster of these clans made up a basic community whose members claimed one lineage. This claim had implications for identifications with each other and helped for the protection and rights of each member.

In this mode of production, there was a variety of productive relations (such as slavery). Each man had rights to land as a male lineage member of his community. Agriculture and commerce were well developed and there was enough food to feed all and to

35

reserve for periods of bad weather or other calamities such as invasion by pests which were common at the time.[2]

Agricultural development encouraged some members of society to venture into other areas of specialization such as commerce and industry. By c. A.D. 1700 commerce, and particularly the trans-Saharan trade, had reached an advanced stage of development in Kanem-Borno and the Hausa states. In North Africa, Tripoli was a center of commerce distributing splendid leatherworks from the Hausa and kola-nuts from the Asante. Because of the stable agricultural economy that existed, the famous trading centers at the oasis of Ghadames drew merchants from Hausaland and Timbuktu. In East and Southern Africa, too, trade thrived. The main trade outlet of Buganda and the interlacustrine states linking up with the trans-Tanganyikan route to Taboar existed even up to the period of colonial intervention.

Besides trade, commerce, and of course agriculture, some people pursued specialist arts such as wood carving, leatherworks, and healing. The precapitalist economy enabled the development of productive forces which encouraged and prompted specialization in healing and perfected what could be called an indigenous African health care system. This system involved a complex network of all knowledge, skill, and practice, whether explicable or not, used in diagnosis, prevention, or elimination of physical, mental, or social imbalance. It relied exclusively on practical experience and observation handed down from generation to generation, whether oral or written. The indigenous system was the sum total of practices, measures, ingredients, and procedures of all kinds, whether material or not, which from time immemorial had enabled the African to guard against diseases, to alleviate his suffering, and to cure himself.[3] Under this elaborate health care system the concepts of disease and illness were derived from doctrines and principles that were rooted in the indigenous cultural beliefs and practices. In other words, the precapitalist African health care system was consistent with its mode of production. As Vicente Navarro observed, and as I will seek to demonstrate in this chapter, each mode of production had its form of health system relative to the development of productive forces in the mode. Thus, the indigenous health care system was related to the precapitalist mode of production.

Health and Medicine in Precapitalist Africa

In precapitalist Africa, as it is today, health and medicine never were separated from political economy. In fact, it was the nature of the economy that determined specialization in the authentic human activity of healing. The practice and organization of health and medicine also were related to the precapitalist political economy. It is interesting that even in precapitalist Africa, the conceptions of health and a healthy individual were equally as encompassing as that of the World Health Organization (WHO) which defines health as the state of complete physical, social, mental, and psychological well-being. In the health and medical systems of precapitalist African, a healer or medicine man was a

> person recognized by the community in which he lives as competent to provide health care by using vegetable, animal, and mineral substances and certain other methods based on the social, cultural, and religious background as well as on the knowledge, attitudes and beliefs that are prevalent in the community regarding physical, mental, and social well being and the causation of disease and disability.[4]

A good healer was one that provided social, physical and psychological therapy and cure. These often involved an undebatable thorough knowledge and explanation of the cultural, social, magical, and physical environment of the patient. Diagnosis in African medicine included a socio-cultural analysis surrounding the patient's condition so that therapy was occasionally only an avenue of cementing fragmented relationships between individuals or between individuals and offended spirits. By reducing inter-personal friction and stress, suggests Tola Pearce, the balance was probably tipped in favor of the patient's recovery and opposing parties were once again at peace and recovery obtained.[5] Patrick Twumasi and F. M. Mburi have shown that these procedures were true of West African and East African peoples.[6] Though these are merely precapitalist African belief structures, they help to show a remarkable difference between the main emphasis of capitalist and precapitalist medicines.

37

As earlier indicated, the buoyant precapitalist agrarian economy enabled the sustained growth and development of medicine. A variety of health specialists ranging from public health to surgery specialists emerged within this African health care system. There were specialist diviners, midwives, bone-setters, magicians, and healers. Others specialized in charms and amulets for warding off evil spirits.

There were health specialists in each village and city, on a variety of cases such as childbirth, child care, bewitchment, diarrhoea diseases and even complicated cases such as arthritis. Not all medicine men and women practiced full time: only a few consecrated ones did. There was, however, a part-time healer of some kind, a family member, in virtually every home attending to simple everyday ailments such as colds and headaches.

Both full- and part-time healers not only were very knowledgeable about the pharmacopoeia of plants, they had an exact and extensive understanding of the nutritional and practical use of plant and wild fruits. According to Hammond-Tooke, among the Mpondu of South Africa "there [was] practically no plant whose bark, twigs, roots, bulbs, or leaves [were] not at one time and another pressed into service as an ingredient in some magical concoction."[7] What was said of the Mpondu of South Africa can indeed be said of many other African peoples as shown in the works of S. K. Bonsi on West Africa.[8] In fact, some people used not only plants but also animal blood, feathers, oils, beaks of birds, and dung as necessary ingredients for therapy.

The procedure for medical consultation under the indigenous health care system was always determined by the nature and the seriousness of the patient's sickness. In some parts of Africa, chronically ill and incapacitated patients such as lepers and mental patients had to stay with the practitioners until recovery. However, in some ethnic groups, practitioners attended to patients in their own homes. In this case the home of the practitioners had to be near that of the patient to allow frequent visits. A practitioner capable of treating complicated cases always was a person of integrity and high status in his own community. His home was always large enough to allow room for the patients and their relatives who often needed to be accommodated. There were special treatment rooms for patients but they also could be accommodated in the large sitting room of the practitioner, especially when guest and treatment room were all occupied. Treatment of many ailments was done publicly in or outside the practitioner's sitting room.

For acute and non-incapacitating sicknesses, healers were often called to the patients' home. However, it was quite normal, too, for patients themselves to walk over to the healer's home to seek treatment. Problems such as stomachache, childbirth, colds, and accidents belonged in this category. Ailments considered by members of the community to be simple and non-mortal never needed the attention of a specialist. The healer was not even required to examine the patient. Mere prescription by a local healer could be enough. In some cases, especially for children, prescriptions earlier given to a neighbor for similar symptoms could be passed on to another person. Most of these simple cures were administered by women.

Healers in many African communities tended to be adult males. Though a few women healers existed, they were very few in number. Women healers specialized in administering simple cures for child care. The most famous women healers were those specialized in issues relating to barrenness and birth complications. Each community had at least one such woman who was always an aged woman who had reached the age of menopause. She was always surrounded by small girls who helped in administering cures for barrenness. Women healers specializing in cases of barrenness still exist in many parts of Africa.

The place of treatment depended on the nature of the disease. Some diseases only could be treated in specially designated areas of a community. While other diseases were treated in public, others were done in private. Sometimes only one or two relatives of the patient would be allowed on the scene. Complicated cases such as bewitchment could only be treated at a particular time and place chosen by the practitioner. Just as in modern medicine some diseases needed to be treated early in the morning while others could be treated anytime or at a time approved by the healer. The commonest special places used for such treatment included shrines, pools, isolated hills, thick forests, river, deltas, road junctions, and other places deemed therapeutically acceptable to the healer and his spiritual friends. Perhaps these places were more convenient for the healers to evoke the spirits, converse with them, and appease them with appropriate sacrifices. With these done, the spirits were happy and conflicts were resolved and the sick person could become well again. The ancestral spirits which were important in the process of patient recovery presumably would be absent if therapy took place in locations not acceptable to the spirits and the healers.

The African medical system had a well developed and effective referral system. As soon as someone showed symptoms of an ailment, recipes were recommended by some members of the family. When symptoms persisted, a local specialist was consulted. If the local specialist, after trying various medicines and concoctions, failed to ensure recovery for the patient, he referred the patient or his relatives to a more knowledgeable and distinguished specialist. His inability to cure an ailment could result in death for the patient. In every community, healers and their various areas of specializations were known, and this in turn facilitated quicker referral services.

The Use of Health Services

Medical and health services in precapitalist Africa were decentralized. This enabled easier access, and it was possible for all members of the society, including slaves, to effectively use the available medical and health services. There were many healers or practitioners and specialists of all kinds, and as such health and medical services were not scarce. Payment was not a barrier to service. Though not all such services were free, payment was usually affordable. Services for barrenness needed no more payment than the goat which was used or a chicken which would be slaughtered and partly used in preparing the medicine which the barren woman would take. The remnants of the chicken would constitute enough payment for the healer. A measure of millet or corn could also be used as payment. For more complicated treatment that required very expensive ingredients and concoctions, a goat could be required as payment. In parts of West Africa, some treatment procedures involved a cow or cows. The cows were slaughtered and the blood collected and given to the patient to bathe with. The meat of the cow, however, was consumed by the therapeutic community while a substantial part of it went to the healer as payment.

Exchange payment was common. Here a patient who was physically strong but psychologically or emotionally ill could offer to clear a plot of land for the practitioner in exchange for the latter's services. This occurred especially in cases where the practitioner combined the healing art with farming. Other healers operated on a full-time basis and used their earnings from healing to support themselves.

All members of the community had access to good health services, even though access was unequal. To be sure, precapitalist Africa was not a classless society and access to medical care pretty well reflected the distribution of wealth that existed at that time. Beside medical care, luxury was also the style of privileged individuals. Individuals considered privileged were those who had health, power, and prestige (à la Max Weber). These attributes were manifested through larger houses, richer diets, more wives and children, and more extravagant clothing than other members of society. The size of their families could number as high as three hundred people made up of wives, children, and dependents. Their farms were large enough to feed them.

To protect themselves and their riches and to ensure continuity in their most cherished primitive accumulation, these privileged individuals (kings, emperors, and chiefs) often needed protective or sinister medicines. To hold on to their prestige, to be respected and feared, they needed extraordinary power to protect themselves from bewitchment or other evil machinations which could emanate from jealous subjects. Because they had many wives and concubines, they needed medicines or concoctions for strength and vigor which would provide them with the romantic stamina to satisfy their flock of wives and concubines. Medicines for fertility, fame, good luck, protection and the like to be sure were very expensive within the limits of the economy that prevailed. Because these were expensive, not all members of the society had access to them. Only that group on the apex of the social hierarchy could afford these luxurious health and medical services.

If those who merely had access to these luxurious medical services were themselves important, one can imagine the position of those medicinemen and healers who were the producers of the service. These producers were equally powerful and were feared in the community. Their importance in society was due to their

41

expertise. As a result of expertise and skill, they often had a cordial relationship with the top political leadership of the empire and kingdom. In one sense it could be argued that there was a good relationship between the institution of medicine and the precapitalist state. They needed each other at the level of the individual and the group. During interethnic wars which were common at that time, distinguished medicine men and healers were called upon by the emperors or chiefs to prepare the army and protect them against the enemy so as to ensure victory. They also treated the wounded. Medicine men and healers, on the other hand, enjoyed the luxury that freely accrued out of the primitive accumulation enforced by the political leadership.

Indigenous healers also were important because of their assumed relationship with the supernatural. The concept of health and medicine was quite diverse but very much related to the metaphysical, which was the ultimate determinant of an individual's fate. By virtue of their special relationship to the supernatural, some healers were so powerful that they intimidated even political leaders. P. A. Talbot reported that some powerful healers among the people of present day southern Nigeria were power brokers who influenced shifts in power relations between both community groups and individuals.[9] The king of Bonny once confessed his reluctance to punish medicinemen and healers even when they were guilty. Thus, even kings were careful in their dealings with healers.

However, the number of healers and medicine men who wielded great power was very small. There was at most one in every community who could be replaced only upon his death. Traditions and customs made it difficult for many powerful healers to emerge. Distinguished healers had to undergo training for many years after which they were supposedly called by some ancestral spirit through dreams or other ways of communication to start practice. Not all healers, however, who went for training became distinguished medical consultants, with wealth, prestige, and respect.

The position of many medical specialists pretty well approximates Eliot Friedson's idea of medical dominance. Friedson explained that in Western capitalist countries, physicians are powerful and they dominate the health sector because of their expertise and monopoly over an important skill.[10] Critics of

Freidson have over the years rightly pointed out the faults of the medical dominance thesis. They explain that physicians are dominant not just because of their scientific expertise and skill. Their class origin, the class basis of medicine, and the support of medicine by the state are some of the main reasons for this dominance.[11]

Our objective here is not to go into the familiar debate on the professional dominance thesis. Rather it is to explain that in the case of healers in precapitalist Africa their relationship with political leadership often was not as important as their skill or their relationship with the ancestral spirits. Their relationship with political leaders came about as a result of the healer's importance and not that he needed state support as in the case in modern medicine. Their relationship to the ancestral spirits was enough source of power for them to hold all people, including political leaders, to ransom if they so wanted. But healers, in their code of conduct, were prevented from such acts because their relationship with the supernatural was an obligation to provide humble service to the lay community and not to misuse the power to spell evil. Misuse of their medical dominance would make them liable to death, deformity, or loss of the most coveted relationship with the supernatural.

Freidson's medical dominance thesis for the most part would be appropriate if applied within the context of precapitalist African medical systems. His explanation, however, does not approximate the reality and social condition of modern Western medicine in Africa. The social forces which determined the dominance and autonomy of indigenous African healers and medicine men are no longer present in contemporary Africa, where the social relations and modes of production are those of capitalism. The belief structures which existed in precapitalist Africa have now been replaced by scientific rationality characteristic of the capitalist mode of production. It is likely, as Navarro suggests, that the social forces that determine the nature of capitalist medicine will be absent under communism so that the organization of capitalist and communist medicine will be remarkably different.[12]

Though Freidson in his study did not discuss the important issue of the relationship between the modes of production and medical dominance, such a relationship is palpable. For each successive mode of production (slavery, feudal, and capitalist) the organization of medicine is seen to be consistent with both the relations of production as well as the level of the development of productive forces. An explanation that comes from the mode of production argument throws light on the continual existence of indigenous medicine along with Western medicine in Africa. While capitalism has taken hold in Africa since the establishment of colonialism, not all of Africa is capitalist. Some rudiments of African precapitalist modes still exist.

The transformation of societies is usually gradual and an old order may not completely die before a new one is born. In his discourse on evolutions of societies, Marx stated clearly that

> no social order ever perishes before all the productive forces for which there is room in it have developed, and new, higher relations of production never appear before the material conditions of their existence have matured in the womb of the old society itself.[13]

The precapitalist African mode still has rudiments which eventually may be eliminated or transformed. Even in advanced capitalist countries such as England and the United States, Navarro has indicated the existence of several modes.[14] He suggests that at the start of the nineteenth century, European capitalist societies were composed of three modes of production: feudal, simple commodity production and manufacture, and capitalist in its competitive and monopoly forms. Navarro went on to explain that each of these three modes had its own form of medicine. According to him

> the fact that different modes and forms of production may exist within the same social formation does not mean they are unrelated to each other. Rather one mode (and one form within that mode) occupies a dominant position with a decisive influence on the others. The dominant mode is the one which gives each society its overall character (feudal, capitalist etc.).[15]

According to Navarro the United States has several modes which also are represented in medicine. Forms of corporate medicine only show the existence of capitalist relations while

44

cottage medicine shows the existence of the petty commodity form of capitalist relations. Each form of medicine has its own knowledge, practice, and institution which are "clearly related under the hegemony and dominance of the corporate medicine form." Navarro's analysis of the existence of corporate and cottage medicine in the United States throws much light on the existence of indigenous and Western medicine in Africa, and the modes and forms of relations of production prevalent in contemporary Africa. A further discussion on modes of production in Africa are considered by Aidam Foster-Carter, E. Laclau, and J. Taylor.[16]

Conclusion: The Future of Precapitalist Medicine

The indigenous African medical system with its body of knowledge, practices, and institutions has as its greatest credit easy availability and accessibility. Its referral process entailed easy access to services, and was very effective. Profit or personal gains were not prime motives for medical practice. Precapitalist African medicine was holistic and sought to treat individuals rather than their diseases as is now the case with scientific medicine. Precapitalist medicine, however, had profound limitations.

In spite of its biologism, positivism, mechanism, and individualism, modern scientific medicine is able to deal with the deficiencies of precapitalist medicine. The discovery of the germ theory coupled with the invention of antibiotics has promoted the status and importance of modern medicine. It controls epidemics that would wipe out large communities. In his book, *A History of Health Services in Nigeria*, Ralph Schram reported that prior to the advent of scientific medicine, millions of people and communities in Africa were wiped out by epidemics such as yellow fever, small-pox, and influenza.[17] Though scientific medicine is superior to indigenous medicine in many ways, it also has learned a lot from indigenous health systems and there is yet more it will learn in order to make scientific medical systems as holistic as indigenous therapy.

Basically, the foregoing discussion described the nature of society, health, and illness in precapitalist Africa before the gradual penetration of Western Christian missionaries. They brought the gospel carefully wrapped in health and educational services. Their arrival, which was followed with a forceful penetration of colonialism, was to have the most salient effects on relations of production in Africa. It significantly altered the dominant mode of production. Capitalist relations of production were introduced with their associated characteristics of unequally distributed and unequally consumed scientific medicine. Capitalism has now grown wide roots whose side effects have far-reaching consequences on health and other social services in Africa.

NOTES

1. See chapter 5 below.
2. D. A. Ityavyar, "Background to the Development of Health Services in Nigeria," *Social Science and Medicine* 24 (1987): 487. For works on pre-colonial African societies, see Toyin Falola, *The Political Economy of a Pre-colonial African State* (Ile-Ife: University of Ife Press, 1984); Toyin Falola, "African Indigenous Economy," *Tarikh*, forthcoming; and R. Oliver and A. Atmore, *Africa Since 1800* (Cambridge University Press, 1972).
3. World Health Organization, *The Promotion and Development of Traditional Medicine*, Technical Report Series 622 (Geneva: World Health Organization, 1978), p. 8.
4. Ibid., p. 9.
5. Tola Ola Pearce, "The Political and Economic Changes in Nigeria and the Organization of Medical Care," *Social Science and Medicine* 14 (1980): 92.
6. P. Twumasi, *Medical Systems in Ghana: Studies in Sociology of Medicine* (Accra: Ghana Publishing Corporation, 1975).
7. W. D. Hammond-Tooke, *The Bantu Speaking People of Southern Africa* (London: Routledge and Kegan Paul, 1960), p. 34.
8. S. K. Bonsi and D. A. Ityavyar, *The Changing Patterns of African Medicine*, Unpublished Manuscript (Accra: 1986).
9. P. A. Talbot, *Peoples of Southern Nigeria*, Vol. 11 (London: Cass Press, 1969), p. 12.
10. E. Freidson, *Professional Dominance: The Social Structure of Medical Care* (Chicago: Aldine, 1970), pp. 13-14.
11. E. Freidson, *Profession of Medicine* (New York: Dodd Mead, 1970).
12. Vicente Navarro, *Medicine Under Capitalism* (New York: Prodist, 1976). See also David Coburn, G. Torrance, and J. M. Kaufert, "Medical Dominance in Canada in Historical

Perspective: The Rise and Fall of Medicine," *International Journal of Health Services* 13 (1983).

13. Robert Tucker (ed.), *The Marx-Engel Reader* (New York: Norton, 1978), p. 5.
14. Vicente Navarro, "Radicalism, Marxism and Medicine," *International Journal of Health Services* 13 (1983): 184-85.
15. Ibid., p. 184.
16. Aidan Foster-Carter, "The Modes of Production Controversy," *New Left Review* 107 (1978); E. Laclau, "Feudalism and Capitalism in Latin America," *New Left Review* 67 (1971): 19-38; and John Taylor, *From Modernization to Modes of Production* (London: MacMillan, 1979).
17. Ralph Schram, *A History of Health Services in Nigeria* (Ibadan: Ibadan University Press, 1973), p. 217.

FOREIGN IMPACT ON PRECOLONIAL MEDICINE

S. Kofi Bonsi

Introduction

Modernization theorists generally have argued that under-development in Africa can be traced to two major factors: defective cognitive orientation of the people and structural characteristics that serve to obstruct development. On the structural level, communal land systems, rural authority structures, extended family systems, and so forth often are cited as obstacles to development. Affective and cognitive orientation such as parochialism, lack of initiative, and inability to act objectively in any problematic situation also are emphasized by researchers and change agents.[1]

The limitations of these modernization theories have been well articulated.[2] Critics have contended that an analysis of the Third World social formation situated outside a historical context is sterile. The promise of this argument is that the most fruitful sociological explanation of any social phenomenon is grounded in historical material. Mills argued forcefully that our understanding of structural changes, for example, are greatly enhanced when we expand our approach to "include a historical span."[3] Since there are no universal principles of structural changes, we can only understand these changes when they are grounded in their historical contexts.

A meaningful analysis of the developments in precolonial African medical practices, for example, requires a theory that is grounded in historical as well as in colonial experience in Africa. In other words, the historical conditions that have affected the development of African medical practices must be adequately addressed. This chapter argues that precolonial African medicine remained underdeveloped for many years because of colonial penetration. The data for this chapter are drawn from the West African subregion.

The Colonial Penetration

Euro-African contact since the eighteenth century had many implications for West Africa. First, the period of contact with Europeans before effective occupation in 1884 contributed to the underdevelopment of African social structures and practices. As Nnoli has argued, the contact took a devastating "toll on the capacity of the people for rapid transformation of themselves and their environments."[4] By incorporating precolonial societies into the world capitalist system in a subjugated position, the rich political systems and social structures which could have formed the basis for the promotion of indigenous cultures were destroyed. Second, the penetration created new productive economic activities in response to the needs of the capitalist countries. This directed attention away from local creative potentials and resources by concentrating on the procurement of primary products needed by the Europeans. Third, the slave trade with its concomitant slave wars created insecurity, mistrust, and destruction of property. These happenings retarded social and economic progress.

During this time of economic exploitation, European missionaries also arrived and began to establish schools in connection with their religious activities. The health institutions which Europeans introduced were supported by Christian religious teachings. Thus, missions exerted an influence through education and sought change in both spiritual and material values of the indigenous people. They claimed that African practices were incompatible with the educational aims and ethical views of the Bible. Fellowship in the Christian faith demanded complete conformity to the Christian doctrine. This involved a rejection of African beliefs, rituals, and other non-Christian observances which formed an essential part of African medical practices. Missionaries and physicians became the most effective means of conquest and oppression employed by the colonial powers.[5]

As with their more militant colleagues (slave traders and colonial governments) missionaries were not so much concerned with the health status of the people. The prime motive of their activities was to evangelize the people. These activities of medical missionaries paralleled the penetration of the Southeast Asia and the military use of medicine by the French in Vietnam. The colonization effort implied in the "opening up hitherto unoccupied towns and villages to the messengers of the gospel" received massive moral and material support from colonial governments.[6]

The colonial period exacerbated the social and economic underdevelopment of the subregion. Europeans introduced social, political, economic, and educational patterns into the indigenous social formations. Parallel modes of production emerged within the same social formations. Among the most important of these modes was Euro-American medical care. New theories, concepts, and interests which were in conflict with African medical concepts and practices were introduced into indigenous life. Thus, in addition to the destruction of the basis for the creative potentials, the parallel nature of the systems stagnated the precolonial modes, essentially because there were no new inputs of ideas to transform them in a self-sustaining manner.[7] The continuation of the element of the precolonial African medicine, therefore, was restricted.

Colonial penetration established not only political and economic domination, but medical imperialism as well. Colonial administrators claimed that African medicine was a less effective and acceptable therapeutic procedure than Euro-American medicine. Mention of African medicine conjured up the awful image of savages dressed in feathers, engaged in sensational dances, and performing irrational and dubious rites based on superstition and ignorance.[8]

As colonial penetration successfully incorporated and fully integrated these countries into the capitalist system, they became potential markets for the medical wares of Europe. Systematic efforts were made to obstruct the development of indigenous medical institutions. This medical imperialism was perpetrated in several ways. First, Euro-American medicine was held to be superior, and a systematic effort was made to ensure its acceptance and dominance in diverse ways, including intimidation. Second, the patterns of medical care in Europe were exported to satellite nations with the capitalist ideological orientation which promoted the well-being of a few as opposed to the majority of the people.

Third, through the "ragged troussered philanthropist apprentice system in which cheap labor is acquired and craft restriction maintained by the pretence of training," there was a constant drain of talents to Europe where most of the trainees learned sophisticated techniques and engaged in research which was completely unsuitable to African conditions.[9] Fourth, conservatism and craft-exclusiveness which characterized Euro-American medicine produced "medical experts" who opposed the development of other medical alternatives. African medicine was suppressed through medical imperialism and constant claims of the superiority of Euro-American medicine and craft exclusiveness.

Colonial conquest not only incorporated African countries into the expansion and development of the world capitalist system, it also systematically attempted to destroy the salient elements of their cultural heritage. In Ghana, the colonial administration's health policy aimed at liquidating indigenous medical practices from the towns. In the 1920s, Gordon Guggisberg, the governor of the Gold Coast, inaugurated a health care program which included the building of Korle Bu Hospital in Accra. To ensure the success of this program, the governor banned the practice of "native" medicine in and around the urban centers.

The colonial penetration thesis thus becomes a model which suggests that the incorporation of West African countries as dependent satellites within the international capitalist system resulted in the underdevelopment of indigenous medical institutions. As Frank has observed, this process of incorporation has wiped out entire civilizations, and destroyed the cherished cultural practices, as the historical development of the capitalist system has effectively and entirely penetrated the apparently most isolated sectors of the undeveloped world. Frank himself emphasized that

> once a country or a people is converted into the satellite of an external capitalist metropolis, the exploitative metropolis-satellite structure quickly comes to organize and *dominate the domestic economic, political and social life of the people*. (Emphasis in the original.) The contradictions of capitalism are recreated on the domestic level, and come to generate tendencies toward development in the national metropolis and toward underdevelopment in its domestic satellites.[10]

The thesis was premised on the argument that the precolonial societies of Africa, and indeed the Third World, were not static. These social formations had capacity to develop through evolutionary and/or revolutionary processes. But this internal dynamism and the process of continued movement toward higher stages of civilization was destroyed by colonialism.

Articulation of Modes Thesis

The penetration thesis could explain to some extent the dislocations which occurred in Third World social formations as a result of colonialism. However, because of its extreme economic and social determinism in which any absence of development is simply explained as an effect of capitalist penetration, it leaves many questions unanswered. For example, it may not explain adequately how precolonial medicine in Africa had persisted and even expanded in spite of colonial penetration which introduced social and ideological instances that continue to articulate their domination. If we accept the thesis of a consistent capitalist domination, we would have no basis for analyzing the phenomenon of persistent articulation of the precolonial medical practices since the capitalist domination would have suppressed or destroyed the former completely. Hence a more meaningful approach is one which accounts for the articulation of both precolonial as well as Euro-American modes of medical care in West African social formations. For despite the capitalist penetration of the Third World and its continued restriction of development in these societies, elements of the preexisting social forms continue to be reproduced. Hence, contemporary Third World societies should be analyzed more meaningfully from a dialectical perspective. This perspective sees these social formations as those which are dominated by an articulation of both capitalist and precapitalist modes of production in which each is trying to increase its dominance. Although the capitalist mode with its attendant institutional structures has attempted to subordinate the previously dominant precapitalist modes, the historical preconditions for the articulation of the former have discouraged total dominance. Taylor argued that dominance of any penetrating mode is determined by its articulation either by the limits within which this penetrating practice can operate, or by continuing

53

reproduction of elements of the pre-existing practice. In the case of medicine, Euro-American health care was not meant to replace the pre-existing African medicine. Rather it was introduced to promote the capitalist economic exploitation of the region.

During the precolonial period, Euro-American medicine was introduced into the subregion through early contacts with the Near East and Mediterranean coastal cultures. The Portuguese who traded with West African people opened up treatment centers in Benin, Warri, and Cape Coast. These services were expanded during the Trans-Atlantic slave trade with Western Europe and America in the sixteenth century.[11] Licensed physicians accompanied the slave traders to care for their staff at various trading posts and to provide services for the slaves to keep them in good health to attract good returns.

In the colonial period, the colonial governments were concerned with protecting their staff in these areas which were infested with endemic diseases to which they had no natural resistance. The health posts and hospitals which were established provided services for the colonial administrators and their local agents. Thus, the facilities were limited to the government residential areas (GRAs), the mining towns, and plantations. This was done to gain more mineral wealth for the capitalists. The main objective of health care establishments, therefore, was to promote capitalist activities in the economic sector, rather than Euro-American medicine. Because of this restricted requirement, health care systems were circumscribed, leaving a majority of the population, especially in the rural areas, to depend on pre-existing African medicine. Providers of the pre-existing health care resisted conscious attempts to eliminate it from the cities.[12]

Nationalism, which characterized the early periods of the struggle for independence, caused some dislocation in the major colonial institutions and ideologies. The nationalist movements clamored for total disengagement from colonial domination. Capitalist ideologies that were dominant in the state apparatus no longer constituted effective support for the proliferation of the capitalist mode of production in many sectors. Although not much was done to change the colonial medical system, nationalist political activities gave impetus to the articulation of the indigenous health care. Because of the inadequacies of Euro-American health care together with the realization that the pre-existing medical system had great contributions to make, the nationalists began to question the prominence being given to the Euro-American system. Thus, the healers were able to come into the open and began to assert themselves in the 1960s.

Combination of Elements of Modes of Production

It can be seen from our preceding argument that African social formations are characterized by circumstances in which capitalist practices cannot transform existing practices in the social formation immediately. Existing practices constitute structures and forms of ideology which are governed by the continuing expansion of elements of the pre-existing mode of production which effectively restricts total dominance by the capitalist mode. Thus, African social formations can be analyzed or examined by focusing on the articulation of different modes of production and possible combination of elements of these modes through a dialectical process.

The dialectical model argues that we cannot understand a given social formation simply in terms of some set of institutions in and through which individuals are organized; we must understand the social processes, in the course of which both institutions and people are transformed. Social units should, therefore, be studied in terms of "a complex of processes, in which things apparently stable, no less than their mind-images in our heads, the concepts go through an uninterrupted change of coming into being and passing away."[13] In studying the course of social change, we should not only concentrate on the external causes but also the internal contradictions and forces of negation within and around a phenomenon. This dialectical approach is fundamental since it discloses connections between units in the process of change in which they acquire various elements and change their properties.

Basic to the dialectical model are a number of propositions which have been derived from observations of the dynamics of social formations. First, it has been observed that all elements are connected in one way or another. However, these interrelationships are marked by contradictions between and within the elements. Second, there is eternal mutability of all elements of the system and the system itself is not a totality or a complete entity but is characterized by a continual succession of developmental stages each of which disappears sooner or later to be replaced by an essentially different stage "which shares the fate of its predecessors." Third, the given social formation in the process of change tends to assimilate substance from its environment which contributes to its survival and development. Hence, at any stage of its development it contains its own inherent characteristics and other factors which are acquired from its environment which are not originally contained in it. Fourth, depending upon the unique circumstances under which the system is formed, it will inherit characteristics which were not contained in the previous forms. This dialectical negation consists in the fact that something of the previous form is lost and something entirely new is added and becomes part of the new system. Development in this sense consists of more than negating some obsolete features of precious social formations, but implies as well the retention of some of the features of those social formations and the emergence of entirely new features which were previously non-existent.

Precolonial African medicine has taken concrete measures to incorporate some of the elements of Euro-American medicine into its practices. For example, instruction in African medicine is now being organized according to institutional routines of contemporary schooling. In addition to formal classroom demonstration and teaching, healers also are emphasizing research into the manufacture and preservation of medical preparations, standardization of dosage, use of scientific equipment in diagnosis and organization of the healers into strong professional associations that would articulate the healers' needs and demands. By incorporating into its practice these aspects of Euro-American medicine, the contemporary healers have modified precolonial medicine to give it an expanded scope. Thus, the combination has produced a mode of medical care the basic features of which are different from the preexisting ones.

Class Interests and Precolonial African Medicine

Underdevelopment of precolonial African medicine also can be linked to the class nature of Euro-American medicine, and the structure that emerged during colonial penetration in the West African subregion. As we have already pointed out, medical

56

imperialism was perpetrated by the neocolonial bourgeoisie using state power. The medical bourgeoisie in neocolonial social formation continued to espouse the superiority of Euro-American medicine. Deliberate health policies that excluded the indigenous practitioners from making their services competitive with Euro-American health services were pursued. However, the limited reproduction of the Euro-American services coupled with its restricted services to a small segment of the populations especially the higher strata of society created a contradiction that led to the re-examination in the 1960s of the insidious policies that had hitherto relegated African medicine to obscurity.

Colonial penetration with its attendant capitalist mode of production exacerbated class cleavages in neocolonial social formations where a dominant local bourgeoisie had emerged. This indigenous bourgeois class has preoccupied itself with self-perpetuation and entrenchment of its interests and comforts. As Asamoa has pointed out, in Ghana this group represents or serves as junior partners of foreign economic and political interests. The major characteristic of the indigenous bourgeois class is "stubborn protection and devoted worship of foreign economic and political interests and capital." The existence of the class "is closely linked with the fate of multinational economic activities."[14]

This class dominates health boards which formulate national health care policies and programs. Using state power, this class has persistently excluded indigenous healers from officially participating in the national health care system. As Walter Rodney has pointed out:

> the conquest of Asia, Africa and the Americas by Europe, and the consequent assumption of state power by Europeans, led to the virtually world-wide domination of European forces of social organization and scientific systems. Western medicine, like virtually all other things European, received official support while traditional systems either received none or were consciously suppressed.[15]

The emerging medical elite has dismissed persistently and contemptuously the practice of indigenous medicine in Africa.

Imperato, reviewing the controversy over the efficacy of African medicine, stated that

> if quality medical care is understood to mean the delivery of services which meet quality standards established by learned consensus on the basis of proven scientific facts, and delivery of personnel who also meet high standards of training, experience and performance, then it would be hard to envisage a role for the traditional practitioner.[16]

For Imperato, progress in medical care and advancement in quality medical services lie in the upgrading of Western-trained professional personnel and material resources such as hospitals and clinics.

The Nigerian Medical Association, through the public statements of its president and the secretary at seminars, symposia, and in the national daily newspapers, has cautioned that practitioners of African medicine should be discouraged since they are likely to cause more harm than good in the treatment process.[17] The Nigerian Association of Resident Doctors (NARD) once advised the Federal Military Government that "the noise about traditional medicine should abate. It is definitely not a solution to our problem."[18] Thus, in Nigeria, the medical elite consider health care as their turf on which nobody dare intrude.

The emerging medical elite also has come to serve the interests of the higher strata in the society. Special hospitals and clinics have been maintained for the privileged classes, all in the name of efficiency. Thus, another insidious characteristic of the post-colonial era is the class segregation of medical facilities along the lines of the racial segregation of the colonial era taken over by the neocolonial bourgeoisie where the privileged class receives Euro-American medical care. Onoge has rightly observed that the unavailability of Euro-American health care services to the majority by reason of inability to pay or class discrimination is a major departure from precolonial conditions.[19] In precapitalist Africa, a sick person was assured medical attention, however limited the medical knowledge of the practitioners. Thus, the real beneficiaries of continued articulation of Euro-American mode of medical care have been the national bourgeoisie who equate it with "modernization."

The termination of colonialism in the 1950s and 1960s in West Africa left unchanged the imperialistic pattern of medical services. Because there were no structural changes in these erstwhile colonies, capitalism continued to manifest itself. For example, through increasing commercialization of health care, the health professional elite and its parent class, the neocolonial bourgeoisie, continued to protect its alliances with the multi-national health industry in order to perpetuate itself, because as Heineke said, the doctor in contemporary Africa is helpless and useless outside a technology-based urban hospital.[20]

The new nations, therefore, continue to be lucrative markets for the world's largest pharmaceutical companies. It has been estimated that poor countries have taken about 30 percent of the total exports of the world's pharmaceutical industry owned mostly by Americans, Germans, and Swiss. The health professionals and the political elite see importation of pharmaceutical products and medical technology as the most authentic way of promoting health. Fundamentally it accumulates wealth for the neocolonial bourgeoisie as well as the giant corporations at the expense of the health of the people.

In this way both colonialism and post-colonial experiences have prevented the development of a viable indigenous medical institution in order to secure unhindered exploitation of the economic benefits of the expanding health industry in the metropolitan countries. We argue therefore, that the political dominance of the neocolonial bourgeoisie, with its interest in perpetuating the Euro-American medical model that caters for its own health needs and economic interests, prevented policies that would have encouraged the further development of precolonial African medicine.

The expansion in indigenous medicine which began in the 1960s, therefore, could be seen as a reaction to both the challenge of colonial conditions and the neocolonial bourgeois class. It was a response to specific political and economic forces that had been generated by the conflict between the narrow class interest of this dominant class and the alienated parts of society. This antagonism took various forms. First, the monopoly over political power was challenged by a series of military coups. Although the military regimes did not change the structural arrangements, they initiated some policies that took cognizance of the interests of the deprived categories of the society and the potentials of precolonial medicine. For example, Acheampong's military regime promulgated a decree which enhanced the status of the precolonial medicine in Ghana.[21] Second, the political and social awareness that was generated during the struggle for independence gave impetus to social groups to rise and challenge the predominant power of the bourgeoisie in the determination of economic and social policies. The struggles were in the form of "conflicts, clashes, and antagonism between the bourgeoisie on the one hand, the lower classes and social groups, namely the proletariat, the middle and lower strata of the peasantry, the weak stratum of the petty bourgeoisie and the lumpenproletariat, in other words the wretched social elements."[22] The practitioners of precolonial African medicine also began to mobilize themselves into a dynamic group to protect and preserve indigenous practices and to assert the African cultural heritage.

Summary and Conclusion

The incorporation of West African states into the world capitalist system through colonialism initiated a process whereby Euro-American medical practice was propagated during the colonial era. The ascendancy of Euro-American medicine coupled with the policy of craft-exclusiveness led to a systematic repression of the indigenous medical knowledge and practice. The power of colonial governments and their control of political and economic systems brought a new cultural hegemony in the medical sector. Indigenous African health care was controlled through government policy since it was considered part of the native "custom." Since the colonial authorities thought little of African cultures they attempted to eliminate some elements in the interests of making the cultures "modern." Most of the procedures and techniques of African medicine were prohibited.

Since its inception, the Euro-American system has been synonymous with a hegemony which maintains social and political control, and fosters the interest of the ruling class. It has served as the instrument of imperialism. The mechanism by which this hegemony is established is in part through the indigenous medical elite. This elite perpetuates the definitions of the indigenous patterns as seen by the colonialists as inappropriate and ineffective. These definitions have become a mechanism by which indigenous health care and the people engaged in it are discredited and subjugated. Because this medical elite wants to maintain as much social distance as possible between its operation and some aspects of indigenous culture, it often becomes more hostile in its attacks on indigenous patterns than their partners. Through this, the medical profession is able to establish and maintain a "technical competence gap" that helps entrench their dominant class position in society.

The health policies of the colonial and neocolonial administrations, therefore, have established and maintained gross disparities in power and status between Euro-American medicine and the indigenous system. By subjugating the indigenous mode of care to inferior status, the practitioners of Euro-American medicine have been able to establish their hegemony in society. Through its various institutions, the state successfully propagated Euro-American beliefs about the legitimacy of medical institutions, distribution of their health services, and the conceptualizations that make these claims appear both natural and inevitable.

Euro-American medicine and public health become instruments of imperialism. Therefore, the activities of the healers to make indigenous medical system more competitive in the past two decades constitutes a challenge to the medical cultural hegemony which neocolonial conditions have perpetuated in West Africa. The struggle against this domination and monopoly is expressed in concrete measures undertaken to make indigenous medical systems more effective and competitive. These developments should be seen as a dialectical result of forces that existed in colonial and post-colonial social formations. The health care legislation which now focus on the activities of the indigenous healers in Ghana and Nigeria also has been generated not in the arena of values, but in the reality of a struggle among classes and class interests.

61

NOTES

1. D. C. McClelland, *The Achieving Society* (New York: The Free Press, 1961); and A. Inkeles, "Making Men Modern: On the Causes and Consequences of Individual Change in Six Developing Countries" in *Social Change* ed. A. Etsioni and E. Etsioni (New York: Basic Books, 1969).
2. A. G. Frank, "The Sociology of Development and Underdevelopment of Sociology," in *Latin America: Underdevelopment or Revolution* by A. G. Frank (New York: Monthly Review Press, 1969); O. F. Onoge, "Capitalism and Public Health: A Neglected Theme in Medical Anthropology," in *Topias and Utopias in Health* ed. S. R. Igman and A. E. Thomas (The Hague: Aldine-Morton, 1975); D. Offiong, *Imperialism and Dependency* (Enugu: Fourth Dimension, 1980); and J. G. Taylor, *From Modernization to Modes of Production: A Critique of the Sociologies of Development and Underdevelopment* (London: The MacMillan Press, 1979).
3. C. W. Mills, *The Sociological Imagination* (Oxford: Oxford University Press, 1963).
4. O. Nnoli, "A Short History of Nigerian Underdevelopment" in *Path to Nigerian Development*, ed. O. Nnoli (Dakar: Codesria, 1971), pp. 48-75.
5. F. Fanon, "Medicine and Colonialism," in *The Culture Crisis of Modern Medicine* ed. John Ehrenreich (New York: Monthly Review Press, 1978); E. R. Brown, "Public Health in Imperialism: Early Rockefeller Programs at Home and Abroad," in *The Cultural Crisis of Modern Medicine* ed. John Ehrenreich (New York: Monthly Review Press, 1978); and J. A. Paul, "Medicine and Imperialism," in *The Cultural Crisis of Modern Medicine*, ed. John Ehrenreich (New York: Monthly Review Press, 1978).

6. A. Y. Ayandele, *Nigerian Historical Studies* (London: Frank Cass, 1979), p. 188.
7. O. Nnoli, "A Short History," p. 36.
8. U. Maclean, *Magical Medicine: A Nigerian Case* (London: Penguin Books, 1971).
9. R. F. Frankenberg and J. Lesson, "Health Dilemmas in the Post Colonial World," in *Sociology and Development* ed. E. de Kadt and G. Williams (London: Tavistock Publications, 1974); and V. Navarro, "The Underdevelopment of Health or the Health of Underdevelopment: An Analysis of the Distribution of Health Resources in Latin America," in *Imperialism, Health and Medicine*, ed. V. Navarro (London: Pluto Press, 1982).
10. Frank, "The Sociology of Development," p. 10.
11. R. Schram, *A History of Nigerian Health Services* (Ibadan: Ibadan University Press, 1971).
12. S. K. Bonsi, *Traditional Medical Practices in Modern Ghana*, Ph.D. dissertation, Columbia: University of Missouri, 1973.
13. M. Comforth, *Dialectical Materialism: An Introduction* (London: Lawrence and Wishart, 1974), p. 10.
14. A. Asamoa, *Classes and Tribalism in Ghana* (Accra: Ghana Information Services, 1985).
15. W. Rodney, *How Europe Underdeveloped Africa* (Washington: Howard University Press, 1974), pp. 6-7.
16. P. J. Imperato, *African Folk Medicine: Practices and Beliefs of the Bambara and Other People* (Baltimore: New York Press, 1977), p. 81.
17. R. A. Ofodele, "Sober Reflections on Traditional Medicine," *Daily Times*, Lagos, 1980; and B. Ramsone-Kuti, "Traditional Medicine is Harmful," *Daily Times*, Lagos, October 6, 1981, p. 2.
18. I. F. Adewale, "The Nation's Health Care System: Strategy and Tactics for Survival" Presidential Address read at Nigerian Association of Resident Doctors Conference, University College Hospital, Ibadan, September 1, 1984.
19. O. F. Onoge, "Capitalism and Public Health," p. 229.
20. P. Heinecke, "Sickness is Wealth," *The Nigerian Standard*, Jos: April 20, 1982, p. 11.
21. S. K. Bonsi, "Traditional Medicine and Social Change in the West African Subregion," in *Sociological Perspectives on*

63

Health and Nigerian Society, ed. Layi Erinosho (Williamsburg: Third Publication, 1984).

22. Asamoa, *Classes and Tribalism in Ghana*, p. 37.

4

THE COLONIAL ORIGINS OF HEALTH CARE SERVICES: THE NIGERIAN EXAMPLE

Dennis A. Itayvyar

Introduction

Before the advent of colonialism, Europeans had had contacts with Africa, notably through trade. By 1504 a Roman Catholic mission had already opened a hospital at St. Thomas Island, off the Bight of Benin. Modern medicine as we know it today did not exist until the nineteenth century. The first Western physicians to visit precolonial Nigeria were those sent by the Church Missionary Society (CMS) of England in 1850. By 1859 two Nigerian ex-slaves, Africanus Beale Horton and William Broughton Davis, returned from England after qualifying as physicians. They contributed to the development of Western or modern medicine in Nigeria.[1] Before 1860 Christian missions visited the coast of Nigeria, but they did not move to the interior or stay long enough to have an impact on health services. The wealth and national resources of Nigeria attracted British imperial interests. A gradual penetration eventually ended in colonial imposition at the turn of this century. With this colonial intervention, and the development of new forces of production, Nigerian society witnessed a new era.

Nigeria Under Colonial Rule

Imperialism was the midwife of Western health services in Nigeria. It delivered Western health services in three ways. First, through the activities of Christian missionaries from Europe and North America who took the gospel to Africa along with Western or modern medicine. Second, it prompted the acquisition of

Nigeria as a colony. Such organization was most important for the development of Western medicine in Nigeria. Third, the nationalist movements that emerged in Nigeria after World War II exerted pressure on the colonial administration to provide more social and economic services for Nigerians. A brief discussion of each of these factors follows.

Christian Missionaries

The limited role of Christian missionaries in the provision of health services which began on the eve of Nigeria's colonial era was considerably increased during the colonial period. Except for the St. Thomas Island hospital founded by Catholic missions in 1504, there were no hospitals until 1865 when the Roman Catholic Church built the Sacred Heart Hospital in Abeokuta. The Roman Catholic Church had more medical establishments than any other Christian mission in Nigeria (Table 1). Between 1897 and 1960 it had a total of thirty-eight hospitals and leprosariums with a total bed capacity of 2,839 distributed in all regions of Nigeria. That number of beds was three times larger than any other Christian mission in Nigeria. Most of the Roman Catholic health facilities were concentrated in eastern and mid-western Nigeria, in areas such as Nsukka, Onitsha, Ogoja, Calabar, Benin, and Owo. Ralph Schram pointed out that up to 1954 almost all the main hospitals in the mid-western regions were owned and operated by the Roman Catholic Church.[2]

Southern Nigeria had more missionaries, more health services, and a longer contact with people of the Western countries than northern Nigeria. Two reasons account for this, one geographical and the other religious. First, both merchants and missionaries coming to Nigeria landed at southern ports such as Lagos, Calabar, and Port Harcourt on the Atlantic Ocean. Both missionaries and merchants often preferred to stay by or near the coast partly because of the difficulty of transportation to the hinterland. Others were afraid of attacks from indigenes who were opposed to the malicious invasion of their country by rapacious aliens. Second, because the people of southern Nigeria had only their African indigenous religion, which was often misunderstood by the missionaries as "idol worshipping" the people became targets for evangelization by many Christian mission groups from

Europe. The so-called dark continent needed the light of Christ. The situation in northern Nigeria was different. Modern health services were mostly provided by missionaries and so the more missionaries in an area, the more health services were available. The implication of this was the maldistribution of mission health services between northern and southern Nigeria. Religious and geographical reasons, though not the only factors, are nevertheless important in explaining the present inequalities in health services in Nigeria.

Table 1

THE DISTRIBUTION OF MISSIONS AND HEALTH FACILITIES
ACCORDING TO REGIONS OF NIGERIA IN 1960

Missions	No. of hospitals 1960	No. of drs. 1960	Beds 1960	Regions 1960
Basal Mission	-	-	30	North
Church of Brethren Mission	3	10	226	North
Church Missionary Society	7	49	622	East, West, North
Church of Scotland	4	32	328	East, West
Lutheran Mission	1	4	137	East
Methodist Miss. Society	7	36	634	East, West
Nigerian Baptist Mission	5	27	372	All regions
Qua Ibo Mission	5	11	267	East
Roman Catholic Mission	38	73	2839	All regions
Sudan Interior Mission	12	20	595	North
Sudan United Mission	13	73	975	North
Seventh Day Adventist	3	14	137	East, West
United Mission Society	1	4	69	North
Total	89	352	7241	4

Source: Constructed from different sources. Most information derived from Schram, R. A., *History of Nigerian Health Services*, Appendix 6 (Ibadan: Ibadan University Press, 1971), pp. 429-31.

Most of northern Nigeria had embraced Islam for nearly a century before the arrival of Christian missionaries and was not willing to abandon it for Christianity. The colonial state was

67

reluctant to allow Western missionaries to penetrate the north. After fighting to conquer the powerful kingdoms of the north, the colonial state did not want Christian missionaries to antagonize northerners who rejected Christianity. Only in non-Muslim areas such as Benue and Plateau States were Christian missionaries permitted.

Between 1901 and 1914 a compromise was reached between the colonial state and missionaries in northern Nigeria. The compromise was that missionaries initially would concentrate on educational, medical and health care work rather than zealous evangelization crusades which could potentially antagonize Muslims. The Sudan Interior Mission (SIM) and Sudan United Mission (SUM) were the main missions in the north. SUM, formerly the Dutch Reformed Church Mission (DRCM), concentrated its work on the people of the middle belt such as the Tiv, Jukun, and Kuteb. SIM faced the difficult challenge of taking up the heart of the Islamic area of Nigeria such as Kano, Sokoto, and Minna. By 1950 SUM had several hospitals and dispensaries spread over the middle belt towns, such as Ibi, Mkar, Takur, and Vom. SIM also had missionary schools, dispensaries and hospitals at Kano, Sokoto, Minna, and Jos. These remain centers of SIM.

By the end of 1960, SIM and SUM had a total of twenty-five hospitals, dispensaries, and leprosariums, ninety-three doctors and many nurses and midwives in various parts of northern Nigeria. Even in 1990 mission health facilities represented a good part of available health services in northern Nigeria, more especially in the rural areas. The Roman Catholic Mission also had seven of its thirty-eight health establishments located in the northern cities of Kaduna, Okene, Oturkpo, Shendam, Yelwa, Zonkwa, and Kakuri. Though the first modern mission hospital in southern Nigeria was founded in 1865 it was in 1914 that the first mission hospital in northern Nigeria was built in Gongola state by SUM.

The significance of the medical missions in the development of modern health services in Nigeria was not limited to hospitals, leprosariums, and dispensaries. Their role in education and health manpower development was equally important. Missionaries opened teacher training colleges, nursing and midwifery schools and training schools for other paramedicals which were most needed for Nigeria's incipient health care system. Missionaries sponsored some indigenes to receive medical or other education

68

abroad and trained others locally. In the former cases, Barau Dikko and Mara Benson, the first two indigenous physicians in northern Nigeria, received their medical education at Birmingham in England with the CMS scholarship that Mr. Walter Miller obtained for them. In the late 1950s Christian missions opened paramedical schools in different parts of Nigeria such as in the cities of Jos, Mkar, Calabar, Lagos, Ibadan, and Bnugo. Mission primary and secondary schools prepared students not only for admission into schools of nursing and widwifery, but also for the lower level manpower positions such as secretaries and clerks which the colonial bureaucracy needed. In more ways than one, it could be suggested that medical missions formed the foundation of what became the modern health care system in Nigeria, as Ayandele and others have concluded.[3]

There is one curious observation about the nature of health services established by the Christian missions which must interest a student of the history of medicine in Nigeria. At the outset cure was the goal rather than prevention. True, medical missions encountered a high morbidity rate. Their overwhelming emphasis on curing economically, however, was too expensive to become part of a health services policy. The problem of the missionaries was their importation of Western conceptions of health and illness to Africa. In the West, ill-health was considered a biological phenomenon which could be mitigated only by the use of Western medicine by a physician. A corollary of the Western conception was emphasis on medicine, the building of hospitals, clinics, and dispensaries and until recently a blatant neglect of socio-economic factors in the aetiology of illness and disease. Examples of Western conceptions of medicine are seen in Talcott Parson's *The Social System*,[4] David Mechanic's *Medical Sociology*,[5] and more recently in Andrew Twaddle's "From Medical Sociology to the Sociology of Health."[6] This kind of modern medicine was inappropriate to Nigeria's level of development. The measure of success of a medical mission often was couched in terms of the number of hospitals, dispensaries, clinics, and physicians. Though mention was made of preventive services such as immunization, health education, and environmental sanitation, they never were accorded priority. The implication of the kind of medicine and its method of introduction into Nigeria was that curative medicine came to be considered the only appropriate form of health care.

69

From this premise, Western-style medicine was grafted onto the Nigerian indigenous health system in the same way capitalism was grafted onto its economic system. The consequences of Western medicine for the health of Nigerians will be considered later, but suffice it to note that whatever form of medicine was brought by missionaries to Nigeria, it was most significant in two main ways. First modern health services provided very meaningful intervention for diseases such as smallpox which traditional medicines failed to eradicate. Western medicine saved the lives of thousands of Nigerians who would otherwise be victims of smallpox and other epidemics. Second, Christian missions in collaboration with the colonial state laid a foundation (however shaky) for the development of modern health services in Nigeria. In Michael Crowder's opinion, the most important factor of change introduced by Christian missionaries in Nigeria was not so much health services, it was Western education.[7] Education was introduced as a factor that would transform the class structure of Nigeria. By providing education or schools to certain people and certain areas of Nigeria, Christian missionaries perhaps unconsciously were introducing a new element in the Nigerian political-economic chemistry, that is the laying of a solid and clear foundation for a new class structure in the Nigerian ruling class. Some members of this class, like Barau Dikko, Obafemi Awolowo, and Joseph Tarka were trained mostly in mission schools. The mission controlled the schools and their curriculum, thus enforcing strong Western liberal ideology at the grassroots in their classroom instruction.

Therefore, the contribution of Christian missions transcended the religious and health factors most commonly associated with them. As Ayandele has shown, Christian missions, by opening schools and training many Nigerians, significantly contributed to the transformation of Nigerian political economy and class structure. The mention of these contributions is not an apology for Christian missions and their culture imperialism in Nigeria.

The Role of the Colonial State

The first hospital by the colonial state in Nigeria was founded by 1871 when the Lagos center for the sick seamen of the Royal Navy was renovated and converted into a forty-two-bed building.

Two years later an Infectious Diseases Hospital was founded in Lagos for Europeans. In the same year, a section of the prison that was built for Nigerian debtors was converted into a mental clinic. Later in 1879 another forty-bed hospital was built in the coastal town of Calabar. These health facilities were all located in cities and towns near the Atlantic coast. They were only for Europeans and later for the Africans they employed. Indigenous healers were still the major providers of health care services for the population.

Meanwhile, kingdoms of the north such as the Sokoto Caliphate, Kanem-Borno, and Tiv were yet to be conquered. After 1879, a British Army Captain, George Goldie, with a few other officers, tried to add the north to the British Empire. He first conquered the Niger area and made Lokoja the political and commercial center of the north. Lokoja was also the army base for confrontation with the northern kingdoms. They started with "legitimate" trade treaties with Sokoto and Kanem-Borno. The treaties conceded commercial power to government firms such as the National African Company (NAC) which was later named the Royal Niger Company (RNC). Trade and a commercial boom allowed for the establishment of health posts in and around Lokoja for the use of the colonial staff and the army as well as European merchants and travellers.

Trade treaties did not mean colonization. They were essentially trading agreements and did not concede political rights to Europeans. The northern kingdoms, especially Sokoto, Kanem-Borno, and Tiv, resisted colonization up to 1900 when the north was unilaterally declared a British Protectorate. After 1900 Frederick Lugard, a British Army captain, led a northern expedition and (thanks to the superiority of the maxim guns) conquered all the kingdoms of the north between 1901 and 1914. In 1914, the newly conquered territory with its distinct political institutions and cultures was joined with southern Nigeria under one political entity called Nigeria. The colonial capital of the north moved from Lokoja to Jebba and then in 1914 to Kaduna. In each of these towns health care services were provided for the use of the European population and especially the British army and merchants.

Inequality in health services between northern and southern Nigeria also may be explained from a structural perspective. Medicine in Nigeria was a corollary or an appendage of capitalism and so the more capitalist activities were concentrated in any city or part of Nigeria, the more health services were introduced in the same cities. All the health services provided by both missionaries and the colonial state were located at strategic economic centers where there were European traders, miners, missionaries, and colonial stations.

The relationship between capitalism (colonialism) and health services development can further be seen in the case of Jos, Port Harcourt, and Lagos. In 1912, when tin mining started in Jos, a hospital was founded. The same was true of Port Harcourt when work started on its mineral oil deposits. The case of Lagos was similar. Many of the hospitals in Lagos were commensurate with increased economic activities. Later Kano had a hospital because it was a commercial center of inland trade. The final extension of health services to Nigerians also was related to the growth of capitalism. For example, Nigerians were the main source of labor coerced by the colonial government in both construction and mining. The capitalist idea that a healthy body means higher labor productivity pushed the capitalists to provide health services, especially for those Nigerians coerced into mining and construction. With this free labor, a railway was constructed from Kano and Jos in the north down to the ports of Lagos and Port Harcourt in the south. The railway helped in the transportation of raw materials from the interior to the coast and then to Europe.

The provision of health services was only a necessary problem that accompanied capitalist activities. The provision of health services in Nigeria was important only as far as it maintained a healthy labor force which enabled higher productivity and hence higher surplus value and profit for the capitalists. The stage was then set for the penetration of capitalism in various areas of Nigeria which continued paripassu with health services development. This trend continued until the outbreak of World War I. The phenomenal impact of both the first and the second world wars on the development of Nigerian health services is briefly discussed below.

World War I and Health Services in Nigeria

The immediate effect of World War I was to strain the Nigerian health manpower, and the development of health services. Many doctors left Nigeria to treat wounded members of the Royal Army at the war front in Europe. The construction of new hospitals was halted. Established hospitals lacked adequate maintenance and decayed. Of the thirty-six medical officers who left for the war, at least twenty-six died in the war. Hence the war had a devastating impact on hospitals. Those at Ilusu, Opobo, and Badagry decayed during the war and were closed.

Unfortunately for Nigeria, the war time saw the outbreak of various epidemics which inflicted untold pain and agony on Nigerians and other Africans. Schram noted that these "diseases killed more people than the war itself." He pointed out that the problem was exacerbated when the war ended in 1918 and Nigerian servicemen came back. They brought with them deadly diseases such as relapsing fever, gonorrhea, syphilis, and influenza which were hitherto unknown in Africa. Thousands of Nigerians suffered and died as a result of disease. The war left a trail of grief, sickness, poverty, famine, and economic hardships in Nigeria (as well as in other parts of the world). However, the impact of the World War I was not completely negative, especially from the point of view of African nationalists.

The World Wars, Nigerian Nationalism, and Health

Nationalism expressed itself through political associations founded by Nigerians after both world wars with the specific aim of opposing colonialism, preaching the dignity of Nigerians, and their rights to self-rule. Nationalists demanded political and economic independence from Britain. They were strong advocates of more economic and social services such as employment, education, health, and roads for Nigerians.

The end of World War I, according to Michael Crowder, created economic and political forces (such as the demand for certain commodities in the West and advancement and growth of Western capitalism) which transformed the Nigerian colonial economy.[8] The construction of roads and railways aided the growth of economic activities which in turn affected the growth of health services. Health facilities which were abandoned during war time due to a lack of funds or manpower were now constructed (for example, the Lagos General Hospital). New hospitals and dispensaries were again located at Jos, Nubi, Enugu, Aba, and

Ijebu-Ode. Missionaries too revived their health facilities and added many new ones after the war.

A development more significant than the reopening of hospitals was the founding of a Dispensary Attendant School in 1920. The attendants were Nigerians trained to assist doctors and nurses in hospitals and dispensaries. The colonial state also followed this with the Yaba Medical School which was to train assistant doctors. These two schools were important in the development of Nigerian health manpower. The first graduates of the Yaba Medical School, such as O. Obasa, later qualified in England as physicians, and came back to Nigeria to give an additional impetus to the nationalist movement which was becoming popular. Physicians such as Barau Dikko were leading members of nationalist movements. These movements encouraged Nigerian physicians to fight discriminatory hiring practices by the colonial government. Schram shows that Nigerians who were qualified as physicians were not allowed to practice in government hospitals, except if they were to attend to Africans.[9] Even those hired were denied equal pay for equal work with Europeans. A physician of African or Indian descent was on a lower salary scale than a European, regardless of the former's seniority. Persistent protests to the colonial government by Nigerian physicians for mitigation finally received attention when a panel was set up by the colonial government to review the situation. The panel, after hearing the grievances of Nigerian physicians, still denied their claims. It justified the discriminatory practice that was already in existence. Part of the report noted that

> we do not believe that in professional capabilities, West African native doctors are on par, except in very rare instances, with European doctors or that they possess the confidence of European patients on the coast. Social conditions, particularly in Southern Nigeria, where European officers live together and have their meals in common under the mess system, and in Northern Nigeria where a larger population of the European staff consists of officers of the Regular Army makes it extremely undesirable to introduce native medical officers in those protectorates . . . in hospitals where patients are practically always natives, it may be

desirable to employ a native doctor, but such cases may be regarded as exceptional, and may be left to the discretion of the local governments . . . if they are employed, they should be put in a separate roster and European officers should in no circumstances be placed under their orders.[10]

African physicians everywhere were outraged by the recommendations of a panel they had hoped would be more sympathetic. This outrage was clearly evident in a release by one angry African physician who sharply reacted against the panel's recommendations:

The Europeans frequently scheduled to serve the British government have almost invariably been of that cheap trashy hide of human extraction, who being incapable of more than the meanest possible livelihood in their own country, have now and again been inflected on West Africa. Godless white men, some of them the veriest heathen, who go to our country to teach vice, inebriety and all the follies of their vaunted Western civilization. We regret the recommendation did not exclude English doctors from attending West Africans. This would, of course, simply give official confirmation to the accepted rule of English physicians refusing to attend the natives (except at hospitals), prevent their get-rich-quick fee, and save some of my people from some of those frightful alcohol sodden spectres which sometimes terrorize their bedside.[11]

Nigerian physicians were equally bitter and staged demonstrations against the panel which denied them parity with European physicians. They argued that to "allow us to run hospitals with African or native patients if we are not considered competent to treat Europeans would only be to expose African population to our incompetence, if such was the case." This unwarranted provocation, according to Nigerian physicians, was to be solved only politically via nationalist movements. When nationalist movements were finally formed, explains G. O. Olasanya, physicians became staunch members.[12] They saw

75

politics as the appropriate terrain for economic and social liberation from the oppressive and rapacious colonialists. In fact, none of the thirty-five graduates of the Yaba School of Medicine became a full-time physician after graduation. Beside the nine who worked for the colonial government, the rest combined private with nationalist political activities.

Nationalism continued to grow and wax stronger and stronger until the outbreak of World War II. This war did not have as devastating effect on Nigerian health services and the Nigerian economy as did World War I. This was because of the European and Pacific focus of the war and the nature of British involvement. World War II actually enhanced Nigeria's economic development because Nigeria emerged from the war with unprecedented prosperity and potentialities for growth and development. The capitalist mode of production had been introduced forcefully from the beginning of the colonization of Nigeria and was now in the process of consolidation. Nigeria's natural resources such as rubber and tin became commodities in high demand on the world market. In Jos, for example, tin mining activities were intensified. Health services also increased as a new sixty-two-bed hospital was opened at Barkin-Ladi near Jos for the use of tin miners. The nearby hospitals at Jos and Kafanchan were also expanded to meet the needs of European staff as well as the over 30,000 conscripted African laborers. There were similar expansions of health services in many other economic centers such as Lagos, Ibadan, Enugu, and Port Harcourt. The target of these health services, however, was the Europeans and the Africans they employed.[13]

Though important, it was not the growth of modern health services but the economic transformation that Nigerians valued most as the impact of the wars. Some scholars have pointed out that the intellectual support given to the nationalist movements by Nigerian ex-servicemen (who had fought in the war on the side of Britain) was also important. Living and suffering pain and frustration together with Europeans in the war was important for Africans because, according to Schram, it helped them to completely abrogate the African myth of "white supremacy." If whites were human beings who like Africans were subject to pain, death, and frustration, then it was time to challenge all Africans to come to grips with the irrationality of an oppressive and rapacious alien governing them and directly controlling their economic and political life. Nationalists believed that people, whether black or white, were the same and had the same abilities. These ideas provided new energy to Nigerian nationalism which had become a political force which the colonial government could not ignore.

Nigerian independence did not follow immediately after World War II, but nationalism was yielding results. The colonial state first had to respond to the major political and economic contradictions engendered by the growth of colonial capitalism as well as nationalism. One response was the decision to extend modern health and educational services to all Nigerians. Nigeria was now at the verge of having a health care system: a ten-year health development plan (1946-56) was announced in 1946; University College, Ibadan, with a medical faculty was founded; and nursing and midwifery schools were opened. All of these were very important developments relating to health services. Evidence weighs heavily in favor of the argument that by establishing such social infrastructure, the colonial state was attending more to the needs of colonial capitalism than to the direct demands of nationalists.[14] With the high incidence of disease and death, it was no more profitable for the colonial capitalist to ignore the need for a healthy skilled labor force. Most of these social services were consumed by both foreigners and indigenes employed by colonial capitalism in Nigeria. After a long struggle the University of Ibadan opened in 1946. A Faculty of Medicine was specifically included to improve the development of health manpower. Many training schools for nurses were opened and by 1960 there were thirty-two nursing and thirty-three midwifery training centers in Nigeria. The two schools of pharmacy at Zaria and Yaba were also important in training junior pharmacists for hospitals. Both government and mission hospitals had programs for training paramedicals such as laboratory technologists.

However, it was the Ten Year National Health Development Plan issued in 1946 by the Director of Colonial Medical Services, Dr. J. Harkness, and his deputy that completely revolutionized the history of health services in Nigeria. The plan projected the building of new hospitals, rural health centers, and nursing training schools (Table 2). It was during the plan period that a Ministry of Health was founded and health services became coordinated by one body. According to Pearce, a health plan for Nigeria was a good idea but the 1946 plan was deficient.[15] She

77

attributes the deficiency to the fact that physicians, Dr. J. Harkness and his deputy G. B. Walker, lacked the requisite skill and information needed for the task. While Pearce's criticism was correct, we should also note that the plan was completely based on the Western conception of health and illness in which the planning of health services was taken to be synonymous with the building of hospitals, dispensaries, and medical schools. On this issue the plan was clear, when it stated that "the first objective [was] the establishment of one or more first-class hospitals in each province with full facilities for the scientific investigation and treatment of diseases."[16] There was clearly no debate as to the need for more hospitals in Nigeria in 1946. But from the overall emphasis the document accorded to curative medicine, there was little salutary potential effect on Nigeria.

Of the estimated capital expenditures on health in 1946, over 67 percent was for hospitals and only 2.7 percent was for rural health centers (Table 2). There was nothing budgeted specifically for immunization, sanitation, health education or other preventive services. While the plan was not completely oblivious of preventive and primary care, there was incongruity between what it said of preventive services and its budget estimates.[17] The colonial government at that time had launched a veritable crusade that was located strategically around the slogan of preventive medicine. This slogan operated only at the realm of rhetoric and hardly any money was voted for preventive health services (Table 2). About 70 percent of the reported and unreported cases of death at this time were due to disease that could have been prevented. Life expectancy was as low as thirty-eight years and the infant mortality rate was as high as 400 deaths per 1000 population. Even in Lagos the infant mortality rate was as high as 228 in 1945 (Table 3). A closer look at the 1946 plan reveals even more limitations. It was an exclusive work by two physicians employed by the colonial state. Personnel outside of the health sector were not consulted. Such an approach was arrogant and was perhaps rooted in the belief that since physicians know about health and medicine, they would be better health planners. This error was clearly demonstrated in the gaps and limitations of the document which was supposedly a blueprint for the Nigerian health care system.

Table 2

ESTIMATED CAPITAL EXPENDITURE ON HEALTH, 1946

| | Estimates of capital expenditure | |
	(in millions of Naira)[1]	%
New hospitals	4.9	67.0
Staff housing	1.7	23.0
Rural health centers	0.2	2.7
Maternity hospitals	0.03	0.8
Pharmacy school	0.2	2.7
Nursing schools	0.04	0.5
Health visitor schools	0.02	0.2
TB sanatoria	0.09	1.2
Mental hospitals	0.06	0.8
Totals	7.3	99.0[2]

Source: "A Health Program for the Nation," *Bulletin of Nigerian Medical Association* (Lagos: Okwesi Press, 1966), pp. 148-49. The last column on the right was computed by the author.

1.   The estimates originally were stated in pounds but for the sake of clarity they are converted to Naira.

2.   The percentages do not total 100 because of approximations.

As physicians, Harkness and Walker were limited in their knowledge of the politics and economics of social services which were both crucial for the task they were to accomplish. They disregarded the politics of resource allocation and were completely insensitive to the distinct regional and ethnic groups of Nigeria. The result was devastating in that a preponderance of health services, hospitals, and rural clinics were located in southern Nigeria. The maldistribution of health services was not only on regional and ethnic levels, but on a rural level as well; even in regions of the south where health services were proportionately more available than in the north, rural areas for the most part were neglected.

Table 3

SOME INDICATION OF HEALTH STATUS IN LAGOS
FOR SELECTED YEARS 1900-1960 (rates/thousand)

Year	Birth	Mortality	Infant mortality
1900	-	-	450
1909	42.2	37.2	315
1920	35.5	28.8	285
1924	32.2	26.9	236
1930	28.6	16.5	129
1935	26.3	13.9	129
1940	29.3	22.5	135
1945	45.0	23.3	228
1950	55.9	16.2	86
1955	46.6	12.4	81
1960	55.8	13.6	77

Source: Annual medical reports of Nigeria, 1930-1960. From 1940-1960 all parts of Lagos are included.

Hospitals and dispensaries were planned only in urban and semi-urban centers such as Lagos, Enugu, Kano, Kaduna, Jos, and towns such as Makurdi and Sokoto. It was only after the 1950s that fortunate rural areas started to have dispensaries within a radius of 100 miles. Such dispensaries often had to serve about half a million people.

It may be poor science to simply explain away all the gaps in the 1946 health plan on the professional and intellectual limitations of Harkness and Walker. To insist on that would obliterate the class factors that may have affected the 1946 plan and exonerate Harkness and Walker as agents of a social class. What we may perceive as gaps and shortcomings of the plan may have been designed by the colonial government to serve political and class interests. Politically, capital health expenditures would satisfy the vocal nationalists, most of whom were in cities, and as such direct

80

beneficiaries of the 1946 health reforms. The new hospitals, clinics, and dispensaries would serve the needs of European traders and colonial bureaucrats as well as bourgeois nationalists. The labor force in cities, especially those employed in mines and those in governmental offices, would benefit from it, thus a healthy labor force would be assured. The direct beneficiary of the 1946 health plan (not surprisingly) was its maker, colonial capitalism, and those it employed (that is clerks, secretaries, and agents). It is entrenched in the first health plan for Nigeria and still contributes to the health services inequalities in contemporary Nigeria since it is the same structure of planning adopted by the post-colonial state.

Pearce is right to assert that the 1946 health plan remains one of the most significant developments in the history of Nigerian health services, because it was the first time health services became coordinated. Health services provided by missionaries, companies, and government were all articulated under what correctly may be called a health care system, that is a coordinated and an organized chain of health services planning and delivery. The combined forces of nationalism and capitalism contributed to the rise of a health care system for Nigeria. Health services became available not only to Europeans and Africans they employed, but to other Nigerians as well.

Finally, it is important to know some of the popular reactions to Western scientific medicine in the early years after its introduction to the Nigerian public. Because modern medicine was new to Nigerians, their reactions to it would have policy implications. Such is the justification for the discussion which will now follow.

Popular Reactions to Western Medicine

Initial reactions to the new health care system were mixed. Some people opposed it, others accepted it with suspicion, and a few others considered it a panacea for ill-health in Nigeria. The main opposition was political. Many Nigerians associated the advent of Western medicine with the oppressive characteristic of the colonial system. They hated colonialism and its forced labor, taxes, and cruel laws. The hatred did not spare all that colonialism had offered including Christianity, schools, and hospitals. That is why many Nigerians boycotted hospitals, schools, and other colonial institutions. Contrary to what some Western anthropologists, such as Alan Burns who shares the colonizers' contempt for the African past may say, Nigerians were not just in a political frenzy of ethnocentric arrogance. Not because of ignorance, irrationality, or unscientific beliefs did Nigerians resist, an anthropologists such as Paul Bohannan would like to explain, but because they opposed modern medicine on the grounds that it was connected with a chain of colonial oppression. To them, whatever was white or Western was oppressive. Certainly the preservation of Nigerian culture was also an important reason for opposition.

The idea of the colonialist nature of health care was reflected in the actions of Nigerian traditional healers. To them the advent of Western medicine in Nigeria was a calculated plan by the white invaders to put them out of healing practice and erode the prestige which indigenous healing attracted. Though waves of oppression kept many people away from modern health facilities, others used both indigenous and Western systems in an attempt to maximize their chances of recovery from sickness. Because many Nigerians refused to visit hospitals and dispensaries or to use the white man's medicine, the colonial state initiated an aggressive legislation against indigenous healers. As was the case in the 1950s those found dealing in traditional healing practices such as the Sopona cult in Yorubaland were prosecuted. Nigerian physicians, however, were pleased with the law that outlawed traditional healing practice because the absence of such healers in cities assured them of enough patrons at their private clinics. Even when they fled to the rural areas to avoid the wrath of the colonial state and persecution from physicians, traditional healers encountered another challenge, one from Christian missionaries who were penetrating the rural areas with the gospel.

Christian missionaries were opposed resolutely to all forms of indigenous healing. They equated indigenous healing practices with idolatry, perceiving indigenous healers as devils-incarnate. Consumers of indigenous medicine were seen as servants of the devil. To avoid indigenous medicine and healers, Christian missionaries provided modern health services such as hospitals and dispensaries in many of the places in which they introduced the gospel. The extent of the involvement of Christian missionaries in medical work in Nigeria is impressive (Table 1). Even today some Nigerian Christians remain hostile to indigenous medicine and believe that a good and decent Christian is one who, among other things, avoids to use of indigenous medicine and healers and who generally show hostility to many aspects of African culture. Christian missionaries in many ways were agents of cultural imperialism in Nigeria.

The reactions of Nigerians who accepted modern medicine were equally mixed. One issue centered on the fundamental tenets of the physician-patient relationship and how medicine could be consumed in the manner akin to that in the West. The physician-patient relationship which Parsons tells us is one of mutual trust and confidence in the West was not so in Nigeria. It was a relationship of profound distrust and tension. According to Schram, Nigerian patients distrusted colonial institutions, and often considered clinical diagnostic questions by colonial physicians as interrogations and had to respond tactfully. Nigerian patients also hated undressing in doctor's officers for clinical examination. To avoid this, which according to Franz Fanon, was generally felt to be a form of oppression.[18] Nigerian patients preferred to consult private Nigerian physicians or even quacks who required minimal or no physical clinical examination for diagnosis and prescription. Nigerian patients could demand and receive an injection or drugs of their choice from private physicians and quacks but this was never the case in government and mission health centers where European doctors presided.

Nigerian physicians made money from this situation as the majority of people preferred private services to government hospitals. In big cities such as Lagos and Ibadan private medical practice became a booming business enterprise. Even physicians employed by the government were attracted to the possibility of the get-rich-quick philosophy that was apparent in private practice. To gain additional income, these practitioners often obtained a part-time appointment with a commercial firm, establish surgeries or clinics in a whole area and some doctors made a succession of tours giving injections virtually on demand, with minimal or no clinical examination, and charged high fees which were often forthcoming because of the unusual faith people placed in the needle. Nurses, midwives and persons who had had the privilege of working in a hospital or dispensary did the same sort of illicit injections for money. This was in contradiction to the precolonial period when healing was seen by many indigenous practitioners as a call for service, rather than a money-making venture.

This crude form of doctoring during the colonial period had its fatal consequences. In 1949 the Sydney Phillipson committee was set up to study the medical situation and make recommendations to the government. Phillipson noted one case in which thirty-five individuals all died after such an injection tour. While not banning private practice, the committee recommended restrictions on injections. Injections were now to be given only on hospital and dispensary premises.[19] However, this law was not enforced. Illicit sale of drugs, and injection tours remain a common characteristic of the Nigerian medical system to this day. The reason may be that apart from missionary and philanthropic physicians, the practice of Western medicine was introduced in Nigeria as a commercial enterprise where doctors, nurses, and other health staff were business entrepreneurs.

Conclusion

The Nigeria of 1861 and 1960 were radically different. Politically, Nigeria became one unit by 1914 and power shifted from the hands of indigenous kings and chiefs to colonial administrators. As the precapitalist mode changed to the capitalist mode of production, significant changes were made in the area of health care. Hospitals and clinics, which were colonial inventions in Nigeria, became important in fighting deadly killers such as smallpox and malaria. Health problems, however, remained and perhaps increased with the advent of colonialism. As smallpox subsided, malnutrition followed in some parts of Nigeria because the structure of Nigerian agriculture had changed to reflect colonial interests. Grazing and farming lands were turned to cash production. Food crops such as yams and cassava gave way to the production of cash crops such as rubber and coffee. Men and women in some parts of Nigeria were coerced into the imperial labor force leaving behind the old and unhealthy who could not satisfy family food needs. Malnutrition was ushered into Nigeria.

Economically, colonialism introduced new productive relations and first encouraged the growth of capitalist productive forces. The combined efforts of Christian missionaries and the colonial government established schools and colleges whose graduates were to be used in the service of imperialism in Nigeria. Some of the Nigerians who were trained in the colonial educational system later became nationalists to fight for Nigeria's independence. When independence was granted on 1 October 1960, these nationalists became part of a Nigerian ruling class whose members control the postcolonial state.

Geographic, ethnic, and class maldistribution of health services was on the list of nationalists as they fought for Nigeria's independence. As a political entity of three regions by 1953, Nigeria's health resources were unequally distributed geographically. For example, the two southern regions had 350 doctors in 1960 while the northern region which had a larger population had only 208 physicians. If self-rule was granted, nationalists had vowed, modern health services would be made easily available to all Nigerians regardless of ethnic, regional, or class affiliations.

In taking their oath of office, the indigenous members of the state at both federal and regional levels reiterated their wish to make health, education, economic, and other services available and accessible to all Nigerians. However, studies by several Nigerian scholars in the mid-1980s showed that inequalities in health, social, and economic services still persisted.[20]

NOTES

1. Beale Horton, *A Treatise of the Guinea Worm*, and *The Physical, Medical and Metrology of the West Coast of Africa* (London: Longman, 1867). Their major contribution was in medical publications.
2. Ralph Schram, *A History of Nigerian Health Services* (Ibadan: Ibadan University Press, 1971), p. 340.
3. J. E. Ayandele, *The Missionary Impact on Modern Nigeria 1842-1914* (London: Longman, 1966).
4. Talcott Parsons, *The Social System* (New York: Free Press, 1951).
5. David Mechanic, *Medical Sociology: A Selective View* (London: Free Press, 1968).
6. A. Twaddle, "From Medical Sociology to Sociology of Health" in *Sociology: The state of the Art* (London: Sage, 1982).
7. Michael Crowder, *West Africa Under Colonial Rule* (London: Hutchinson, 1968), p. 372.
8. Crowder, *West Africa*, pp. 482-505.
9. Schram, *A History*, pp. 181-215.
10. G. C. Denton, *Observation of the West African Staff Committee Report to the Secretary of State dated July 26, 1909*, no. 27556 Colonial Office 1901 and no. 158 Gambia office.
11. Edward Mayfield Boyle wrote the letter from Washington. Cited in Schram, *A History*, p. 138.
12. G. O. Olasanya, "The Nationalist Movement in Nigeria" in *Groundwork of Nigerian History* ed. O. Ikime (Ibadan: Heinemann, 1980).
13. Schram, *A History*, pp. 133-249.
14. Bade Onimode, *Imperialism and Underdevelopment in Nigeria: The Dialectics of Mass Poverty* (London: Zed, 1982).

15. Tola Pearce, "Political and Economic Changes in Nigeria and the Organization of Medical Care," *Social Science and Medicine* 14 (1982): 90-98.
16. J. A. Harkness and G. D. A. Walker, "A Health Program for the Nation" in *National Bulletin of Nigerian Medical Association* (Lagos: Okwesi Press, 1966).
17. Ibid.
18. Franz Fanon, *The Dying Colonialism* (New York: Grove, 1963).
19. S. Phillipson, *Report of a Commission on the Private Practice of Medicine* (Lagos: Government Printer, 1949).
20. See S. O. Alubo, "Underdevelopment and the Health Care Crisis in Nigeria," *Medical Anthropology* (Fall 1985): 320-35; Ngimiro Ikenna, "Militarization in Nigeria: Its Economic and Social Consequences," *International Social Science Journal* 35 (1983): 125-40; Dennis Ityavyar, "Health Services Inequalities in Nigeria." Unpublished manuscript, Department of Sociology, University of Jos, 1986; and Toyin Falola, "The Health Component of the Underdevelopment Crisis," mimeo, unpublished paper.

5

THE IMPACT OF COLONIAL RULE ON HEALTH DEVELOPMENT: THE CASE OF KENYA

F. M. Mburu

Introduction

The recent history of Africa has been influenced largely by European colonial powers. Colonial history has affected the socio-economic institutions, structures, social philosophies and perceptions of African societies both from within and without. Kenya, like other former colonies, has not been immune from the diverse forms of domination through conquest. Her institutions have been shaped accordingly, sometimes by way of protest and sometimes by way of positive response to colonial penetration. The thrust of colonial domination was to mold systems in the colonies which were appropriate to socio-economic patterns arising from the particular development situation of the relevant colonizing power. Socio-economic analysis of both colony and metropolis shows a developmental pattern underlying race relationships or political structure in the colonies. This chapter focuses on one of the major social institutions—health—and shows the determinants of history on the health systems of today.

Broadly speaking, the development of human societies is affected by four closely intertwined human activities: political, socio-economic, cultural, and medical. In this chapter I have taken the term "medical" to refer to the ideology governing the concepts of health and disease. From these four human activities the strongest and most far reaching is the political. Political activity determines the magnitude and the direction of the others. Socio-political history demonstrates that the principal determinant of the welfare of the population in Kenya during colonial rule was the thrust of colonial conquest. This chapter further shows the influence of political economy on the health system in Kenya.

Areas of Colonial Conquest

In Kenya, colonization started about the end of the nineteenth century and quickly affected the four broadly-related areas mentioned above. In the political sector, indigenous ethnic groups and their systems of government were subjugated under a newly-imposed system. Instead of paramount chiefs and elders of the clans, a complicated network of "rulers" was instituted, starting with an imposed chief, district and provincial commissioners, and culminating in a governor. The tribal council had to give way to a council of ministers, and later to a parliamentary system, from which the indigenous peoples were excluded. In this way there was total exclusion of Africans from the arena of self-determination. Decisions were made by others on their behalf. This absence of political rights was the basis for other areas of expropriation, for the indigenous populations could do nothing without political power.

Similar kinds of socio-political systems were found in many former European colonies including Mozambique, Angola, Zaire, and in the former British colonies of Zambia and Zimbabwe. Colonial rulers may have been different, but the outcome of colonial domination was invariably similar.

Regarding economic activities, colonial domination changed the existing modes of production and distribution of benefits, and reversed the rationale for economic activity. Formerly, people paid themselves for their own welfare. Under British colonial rule, however, the rationale of production and the associated economic activities and results were for the benefit of the citizens of the United Kingdom. Without exception, this rule applied in all colonized societies. The African populations were used (and are still used notably in South Africa) as a cheap means of profit-making for European entrepreneurs. The laborers were not citizens comparable to European immigrants. On the contrary, they were relegated to the lowest rank in a two or three-tiered socio-political system. In Kenya, for instance, Europeans were at the top of the structure below which were Asians and further down Africans. As would be expected, the pyramidal structure had a wide base of

Africans and a sharp apex of Europeans, colonial officials, farmers, businessmen, and professionals. The colonized people were not citizens, although some of them had died during two world wars.

Cultural domination destroyed or attempted to destroy African ways of life, religions, social assimilation patterns, and customs. The pulpit, for example, was used to spread words of Christian love and justice; sometimes it condemned sacred customs integral to African life. Notable among these antagonistic areas was the Agikuyu practice of female circumcision and related ceremonial activities. Kenyatta's famous defence of female circumcision in the early 1920s became a rallying point in the struggle for independence. In Uganda, for instance, the Baganda expected a well-brought up future bride to have manipulated and elongated labia minora for the purpose of strengthening future marital sexual bonds. The custom was not spared condemnation by European religious leaders. It was argued that the custom was primitive and immoral. Europeans rarely understood African customs. Similarly, other customs and beliefs were subject to attack. Even today, African forms of prayer often are regarded as the glorified work of evil spirits at best or of Satan at worst.

In the medical field, colonial domination followed the pattern of the other three. Indeed they prepared the ground as it were in which this last would flourish and set the tone for the existing health care system.

No society has existed without a health care system that endeavored to cope with social, psychological, economic, and physical ills or areas of disharmony. The traditional African health system is perhaps best known for the maintenance of some established balance between the individual and the community on the one hand, and the surrounding environment on the other. In this equation is included the spiritual realm. The practice of this traditional health system was unique in many respects, especially in the interactions between the patient and the doctor and the patient and the family. While the doctor may be a recognized specialist, the "feeling-lessness" and detachment, characteristic of modern health care systems, did not exist. In most cases, the doctor was known by either the patient or the members of his clan. Of necessity, with a few exceptions, the traditional doctors shared the belief system of the patient. Indeed, the doctor and the patient belonged to the same integrated socio-cultural group supported by an established framework of social norms. This last aspect probably explains the high prescription compliance rate in traditional health systems.

The medical care system existing today was entrenched in Africa partly as a direct attempt to suppress traditional African systems (including health) and partly, and more important, as a necessary condition for colonial "stewardship of dependent peoples." Even today modern medicine in conjunction with other modern institutions attempts to show that most aspects of traditional medicine are detrimental. When the modern medical system was established it was believed that a minimum standard of health of the "natives" was a necessary condition for the African to be able to provide minimum work performance in whatever assignments were given him. Furthermore, the health of the European settlers was indeed partly dependent on the health of the natives. The danger from communicable disease of which the European had built no immunity was always present. The use of malaria, cholera, and blackwater fever as a common "deux ex chanina" in nineteenth and early twentieth century fiction, reflected a very real concern and acceptance in colonial culture. Effective control of such diseases would be limited unless the native carriers were themselves free of the maladies. European employers therefore were advised to invest in the health of their native laborers, for in them lay the very survival and success of the employer. In 1927, for example, the Director of Medical and Sanitary Services, Dr. John Gilks wrote in his annual report that

> employers of labour and township or municipality authorities must realize that the native living under insanitary conditions [was] a danger to the public health of the farm or township and that proper provision must be made for his accommodation under sanitary conditions if the health of the other communities [was] to remain satisfactory and economic progress [was] not to be retarded.[1]

Gilks' recommendation ran counter to the very principle of colonization: exploitation of both the colonized and their environment.[2] The colonial office in London and its local administrative wing had so far found it hard to modify this

91

principle. It was perhaps for this reason that Gilks issued a cautious recommendation regarding the health status of the African laborers, many of whom had died in World War I on the side of the Allies. Insinuating that short-sightedness was endemic among government officials and local entrepreneurs regarding an effective and efficient labor force, Gilks wrote as follows:

> There is now, among many of the more far-seeing employers, a feeling that time is ripe for more definite requirements on the part of Government as to the conditions under which labourers should live and be employed, and almost enough material has been collected to enable such requirements to be formulated. This, of course, will have to be done with caution![3]

Accordingly the then health officials could not even recommend training of Africans. The time was not ripe.[4]

The medical system, vigorously instituted, was designed to benefit the European immigrants. The Africans were just a necessary problem of that maintenance process. Total neglect of the natives was deemed impossible in view of the importance of native labor and in view of the high prevalence of infectious diseases. Medical experts therefore recommended health promotion for populations in both native reserve and settled areas. No section could be neglected in either area without other sections being prejudicially affected.

Understanding of the area of colonialism outlined above and their effect on the current social systems is not only desirable but necessary. Medicine, socio-economic values, political norms and indeed the whole society are closely intertwined. As Stainbrook wrote:

> The understanding of the structures, functions, and values of social organizations is not optional or elective for medicine and public health, but imperative. The sciences of social man and of individual behaviour area an integral part of basic medical science.[5]

The maintenance of any particular system requires that it be partly an articulated regulatory system, partly an established normative system, and that institutions be staffed by individuals devoted to the survival of the system. It would have been completely out of character to have a colonial system run by people who did not believe in the system.

Indeed, in Kenya and other African countries at the end of the twentieth century we see a similar pattern of system maintenance emerging, perhaps more forcefully. With a few exceptions, staffing of many public institutions often is based on loyalty to the system rather than ability to run the system. The health field is no exception. The growth of hospitals thus is a logical development and will probably continue until health system goals are changed and staffed with personnel who believe in the change.

Socio-historical Development and Medical Care

Missionary groups established a foothold in Kenya about 1890. They were preceded by the Imperial British East African Company (IBEA) in 1888. In 1896, colonial domination over Kenya formally was effected. In 1920, Kenya became a British colony and protectorate. This status lasted until 1963 when Kenya attained independence; in the following year she became a republic within the Commonwealth. Since the establishment of formal colonial administration the three establishments—IBEA, missionaries, and the colonial government—closely performed their respective roles more or less harmoniously, though not as comfortably as would have been expected.

IBEA: The Economic Factor

The principal role of IBEA was one of economic activity. This activity required a population with some standard of health. Where necessary, however, the minimum standard was set aside, presumably to increase the profit margin and also because health was not thought to have a direct contribution to profit-making. The medical services of the IBEA were therefore limited to the employees of the company but not their relatives. Quantity and the quality of the services offered progressively declined from the Europeans through the Asians to the Africans. Little attempt was made to reach the

93

rural settlements where African labor originated. This became evident during World War I. When Africans were subjected to medical examination to find out whether they were eligible to join the military activities, 34 percent of recruits from central Kenya were found to be unfit to be porters. Another 33 percent were found to be unfit to be laborers![6] For the general population the prevailing low socio-economic conditions, including housing, sanitation and other environmental deficiencies in a wider environment of malaria, plague, trypanosomiasis, to name but a few, contributed to the unexpectedly high morbidity and morality patterns.

Even though the soldiers, porters, and laborers in the army were the select healthy minority, they lived under harshly subhuman conditions from where they acquired other diseases, such as syphilis and concomitant weaknesses. This was evident during the war. It is said that of the 4300 Kenyans killed in the military 70 percent succumbed to disease. Even the carriers who were supposed to be of a higher health standard were not immune to disease. Of the 350,000 porters, 18 percent died from disease. The newly acquired diseases were taken back to the native reserves where they spread easily. Perhaps owing partly to a poor understanding of epidemiology at that time and partly to resource constraints, colonial authorities saw no need to take any precaution to protect the natives from diseases to which they had no immunity. On the whole, then, what is generally called a "peaceful permeation of Western civilization," was clearly a forceful and brutal, though not necessarily deliberate, penetration of Western socio-economic pursuits into Africa.

A modern system that approximates to the IBEA health service is the occupational health services system, something often beyond the reach of those outside a particular occupation or economic concern. Some organizations such as the armed forces, large plantations, and most industrial concerns provide curative services for their workers and their families. As the manufacturing organizations were generally based in urban centers, the occupation health system, together with other systems, enhances the urbanization of health care. Inadvertently, the gap between the quantity and quality of urban care and rural care continues to increase with economic development.

94

The Missionary Factor

The missionary factor in the development of health services in Kenya has never been doubted. But the relationship between the religious groups and the colonial government is still a controversial issue. It is necessary, however, to look into the contributions of the religious groups and the rationale behind their work in order to understand the current situation.[7] The relationship between missionaries to Africa and European expansionism has been less one of competition and more of complementality. Perhaps the belief common among African intellectuals that the Bible was the standard for the gun is not completely unfounded.

The missionary workers played their cards well to gain recognition and favor among African rulers. Medical knowledge and the art of reading and writing were among those cards. In Buganda for instance, Speke is said to have impressed and befriended the *kabaka* (king) in 1860 only when he made use of his rudimentary medical knowledge.[8] In 1878, the first medical missionary was asked to provide medical advice to the kabaka's palace. By way of reciprocity the kabaka bestowed his own blessing on the missionary and Christian work. By and large such blessing lasted until the kabaka's memory was adulterated by a new curiosity about other missionaries. Father Lourdel, the first Catholic missionary to Buganda, successfully treated the kabaka for dysentery largely to attract the kabaka's attention and to gain the privileges accruing from his satisfaction. As a consequence of medical miracles, the missionaries were permitted to preach and convert in the kingdom.

In Kenya too, healing went hand-in-hand with proselytization. Perhaps promises of spiritual rewards in the next life required precursors in the form of earthly rewards such as health. Both the Catholics and the Protestants recognized health work as a potentially converting element. The missionaries were quick to realize that the praise of the new God and the attempt to banish the old were not sufficient to convince the natives.

Although missionaries opened up outposts in remote areas and larger "health centers" in their more important areas, their impact in the reserves remained low in a few places and nil in most communities. This fact came to light during World War I as

95

noted earlier when the health of most of the would-be military conscripts was found to be less than that which the colonial government expected after nearly two decades of administrative activities.

The second half of the 1920s saw the expansion of both administrative and missionary medical work in response to earlier disappointments. Generally, however, the religious and medical services were made available exclusively to the African and Asian communities. In spite of the initial dubious motives, missionary medical activities were the single most important attempt to influence Africans in their own environment outside the prevailing colonial structure. Missionaries may not have provided quality care but certainly they provided a significant portion of medical services however inadequate in quantity and of coverage.

The Missionary Health Services

Today, as in the past, the missionary health care system has followed the denominational pattern of acceptance and establishment. For example, neither the Catholics nor the Protestants have set up a health facility where they do not have a strong following. The health care facility is more often than not a reward to the community for accepting the church and an incentive for the doubtful to commit themselves. Though theoretically a religious community need not express itself through the physical building of a church, in practice the church building becomes an important and often necessary symbol and base. Throughout the missionary presence in Africa the same pattern has dominated health and education activities. Hospitals and schools are seen as the ultimate realization of health care and education.

The missionary health care system thus has been largely based on hospitals in rural areas. These facilities are better equipped and staffed than comparable government services. The focus of the system has been the provision of basic curative services required in the rural and often inaccessible areas.[9] In such areas only expatriate nurses are available to provide care. The cultural and training backgrounds are not inconsequent to the type of services they emphasize. But the trend currently is changing in favor of community-based care. The resources of the missionaries, however, are often far too inadequate for rapid expansion where they are most needed.

The Government/Public Factor

Within a few years of the establishment of colonial rule, Kenya and its neighboring countries had three distinct racial groupings: European, Asian, and African. The three groups were the basis for the three medical systems.[10] European, Asian, and native hospitals were not established by accident, they were designed to emphasize the fundamental chasms dividing the three radical groups, and perhaps the colonial understanding of balanced development. The colonial administrator became no less a charlatan in political manipulation than in the use of health development. As a rule it was decided that the health system provided to the natives was to be for the purpose of keeping them usable—that is, exploitable—by the European entrepreneurs and civil servants. Not surprising, colonial administrative and economic development, religious expansion and health care growth followed similar paths. Indeed they were inseparable.

Just as there was a three-tiered society, government supported a three-tiered system of health care, each level serving its particular group. There were European hospitals, African hospitals and "Asiatic wards." Later the Asian communities were able to establish their own Asian hospitals notably the Aga Khan in Nairobi and the Pandya Clinic in Mombasa. There used to be European and Asian but no African doctors. The colonial government position was that the African lacked a well-developed brain to learn any advanced work and, in any case, he could not perform tasks independently.

The training of African medical orderlies to staff dispensaries began in 1920 but training of doctors for higher more complex tasks did not start until about 1935. Even then, facilities were limited to a few. The medical graduates from Makerere, a constituent college of the University of London, were very slow in coming. For instance up to 1949, only fifteen graduates had been produced over a period of fourteen years. Even after training, the African medical graduates had to serve under European and Asian doctors. A European graduate was a "medical officer," an Asian graduate was an "Asian medical officer," and the natives were

97

"assistant medical officers." Reports from the latter indicate that the African doctors received discouraging encounters from other medical colleagues, even in the wards. The ward sisters, invariably Europeans, could sometimes insult the African doctor with impunity. Prescriptions ordered by African doctors were subject to changes by the sisters. In addition, the so-called assistant medical officers were discouraged from further training in specialist areas. This largely explains why the current top medical specialists in Kenya had to leave government service in order to specialize.

Public medical services were limited to the urban centers and to those areas considered to have adequately accepted colonial rule. The relationship between the provision of medical services and the administration is not quite incidental. In most cases medical services were the rewards for subservience. In this regard the administration differed markedly from the missionary, the latter using medical services to gain access to the native souls. For the government, however, medicine and politics were seen as the legendary carrot and stick. A pioneering colonial doctor, for example, once said that it was necessary to give "the Native tangible evidence that government is something more than a mere tax collector in justifying his recommendations for increased budget for the health department."[11] Even after the African had died fighting for the colonial Crown, the major causes of death, plague, malaria, sleeping sickness, influenza, and environmental sanitation hazards remained largely untouched. The humanitarian aspect of medicine had yet to reach the African reserves. In addition the introduction of the new medical technology was not accompanied by concomitant changes in living styles. Consequently, the new technology was used to treat illness as presented, without any significant attempt to get the cause of the illnesses. No medical system can be successful if it works in a vacuum where the society which gives rise to the health problems to be controlled is ignored.

It should be noted, however, that the medical department was not free in its own administration. The colonial office in London set out the objectives to be pursued by all departments and at times laid down regulations in respect to the strategies for achieving the objectives. Budgetary inputs were imposed by the colonial office; the department could not alter the budget presented. This was strong leverage on the part of the colonial office.

Racial differentiation was a necessary condition for colonial rule. As far back as 1903, the colonial office specified the objectives of the medical department as, first, to preserve the health of the European community, especially the government officials; second, to ensure that the native and Asian labor force was in good working condition; and third, to prevent the spread of infectious diseases common in the region. Accordingly, there was a greater financial outlay for the Europeans and Asians than for the African groups.

For instance at the mental hospital, the ratio of African to European/Asian cost per patient bed-day was about 1:5 in 1945 and 1946, and about 1:3 from 1947 to 1949.[12] At this hospital, the African patients were kept "in the totally unsuitable prison environment" awaiting vacancies to be found. For the other races, such conditions were never allowed. An instance of the state of the European patient appears in the 1949 Annual Report where it is said that "comfortable and homely furnishings were provided on a scale far more generous than ever before."[13]

The Present Public Health Care System

There exist four main considerations for determining health goals: the individual, the professional provider of care, the government or policy maker, and the community. For each of these health goals are often expressed as demands for action to cure a prevailing or perceived health problem. Health goals may be identical for a number of groups, yet the strategies to achieve the goals are often dissimilar and sometimes contradictory. At the very elementary level, the chosen strategies will be circumscribed by the prevailing socio-political system, technology, socio-economic and cultural values and attitudes towards both the assumed problems and the assumed benefits.

How does one convince an individual patient to "treat thyself" when the problem is seemingly self-inflicted? How can the individual medical professional be convinced that prevention is better than cure when he earns his livelihood by treating the sick? Business lore has it that no businessman should try to run himself out of business. Similarly a community may demand visible evidence of health care such as a hospital even though that may not be what is needed. The same problem affects policy makers, that is the dilemma between providing and supporting glamorous institutions on the one hand, and less politically visible although more practical institutions, on the other.

In Kenya, as elsewhere in Africa, there are always demands from the majority for more and better health services. Such health services are not necessarily the most technologically sophisticated. Only a small minority clamors for sophisticated care. Unfortunately, the minority do not share in either the problems or the perceptions of the majority, most of whom may be poor, illiterate, and politically isolated.[14]

For policy-making purposes the latter segment of Kenya society, comprising over 70 percent of the population, is a numerical majority. History has shown that this majority's choices may be limited by the choices of the minority which has greater political power. What the majority may want is subject to approval by the elite. What the latter want they will fight for and is what may be instituted. If the numerical majority, the rural masses, do not want a large hospital, they will have it anyway. That is the current situation in Kenya. In spite of grandiose rural health development rhetoric, hospital development and maintenance absorbs the lion's share of the health budget. In staff development post-graduate training (specialization) is becoming the norm in a country where the population-doctor ratio is over 50,000:1. Paradoxically, the major health problems and causes of death are largely due to environmental health and socio-economic deficiencies. However, medical education, largely clinical and institution-based, is tailored along standards imported from Britain, even though Kenya and Britain have little in common in terms of health problems. The goal in the medical profession is to produce medical doctors with an international flavor complete with colleges of physicians and surgeons with community-based or primary health care having no place.

Characteristically, the management of the needs and anxieties of the many are controlled by a minority of intellectuals, professionals, business leaders, and not least by policy makers. In this, Kenya is not peculiar; there are socio-political precedents. Were the national resources to be utilized more rationally, the currently available knowledge could reduce whooping cough, tuberculosis, sexually transmitted diseases, urinary track infections and others by up to 100 percent. Nutritional disorders could be reduced by from 70 to 80 percent within five years.

The major reason for current health development trends is a paradox so gross among health professionals, health managerial ranks, and other elites as to be pathological.[15] On the one hand is the increasing demand by the elite for the establishment of what is assumed to be the "best" care available, and on the other is the neglected realization of the increasing need for basic health care services in rural areas. The demands have been especially achieved in urban areas and for the better paid. But for the majority neither the quality nor the quantity is adequate. There is a conspicuous lack of balance in health planning and programming. Reluctant attempts on the part of the elite to reconcile these two demands has led to the existence of a managerial malady which has paralyzed effective health planning and service delivery.

Although the public health system should provide health care equitably to every person, this philosophical goal as specified by the government health plans and international agencies have yet to be attained. The largest and best equipped hospitals are actually "islands of excellence" in urban areas. The current system has grown along the trend established by the colonial system.

Political activities are games played according to curious rules for the main actors vis-a-vis their followers. Social groups are mobilized around some articulated objectives. Once alliances have been successfully established, however, the rationale for political organization often changes: there is no guarantee that the original objectives will be pursued. In some cases, even when pursued, new rules may have to be formulated. At independence the political party, the Kenya African National Union (KANU), was a strongly nationalist party. It collapsed to near-extinction within a few years. Politico-administrative power was transferred from the party and parliament to the provincial and district commissioners, exactly as it was during the colonial period.

African leaders have demonstrated a few failures, among which is their inability or unwillingness to make structural changes in their independent republics. With a few exceptions—notably Tanzania, Mozambique, and Guinea—development philosophies in these republics are largely borrowed from former colonizing powers. Examples are numerous. In 1963, Kenya became

101

independent of British colonial rule. One of the major areas of contention between Europeans and Africans was the inequitable distribution of resources and public benefits. As we have seen, Europeans controlled political debate, instruments of political processes and, indeed, the results. Large tracts of the best land were reserved for white farmers. Most favorable urban residential areas, schools, and other amenities were set aside for whites. Debate was pursued and armed clashes (the Mau Mau war) waged to wrestle those privileges from Europeans and Asians or at least share them equitably with Africans.

But into the shoes of the white man readily stepped the black Kenyans endowed with education, leadership ability, and wealth. Most of these had been the vanguard of the struggle for Uhuru (independence). Since Uhuru, Kenya has been roughly dichotomized into a few who inherited "Mzungu's" (white man's) privileges and consumption habits and the masses who are still outside the former privileges of the white man. For the few, conspicuous consumption habits, exclusive residential areas, schools, and hospitals abound largely at the disposal of a near-exclusive class composed of expatriates, Asians, and a corps of African elite who Frantz calls "Black skins, White masks." The new society has a distinct class character replacing the pre-Uhuru racial criterion for access to privileges. It is hardly surprising then that the colonial institutional structures, including the health care system, exist almost intact.

Indeed there are structural problems, both economic and ideological, which entrench the system. With the unending expansion of hospitals, the more needy rural populations progressively becomes disfranchised vis-a-vis urban populations in terms of the relative significance of rural health expenditures.[16]

The Private Sector Services

The developments outlined above have indeed carried equally into the private sector. This sector consists of two levels, one as large scale and complex metropolitan hospital services operated on the rules of the marketplace. The genesis of these hospitals is related to the historical racial segregation system propagated by the colonial government by which hospitals had been set up to serve European, Asian, or other communities.[17] The system flourished after independence because there was a market among the African elite. These hospitals were, and still are, to be found in the major cities. The second level consists of a host of private clinics of varying sizes and capability, usually owned by one or more doctors, most of whom are general practitioners. The thrust of their practice is curative medicine, mostly in urban settings where the market is large. Relatively few people can afford the services of private doctors, especially the specialized cadre.

As under the economic and socio-political structure of colonial times, the private sector tends to operate on a business basis. Characteristically, specialization is a growing tendency, and is considered to be a necessary achievement in some hospitals. The doctors' specialization requires specialized diagnostic and curative equipment. Consequently the molding of exceptional centers of excellence is already a reality and the norm. Surprisingly, the government health manpower development system, in which specialists are produced at the expense of the public, inadvertently serves the goals of the private sector. The quest for equitable distribution of the quantity and quality of care cannot be met in this manner.

Conclusions

The historical development of Kenya, and in general sub-Saharan Africa, has largely determined the existing health system. Attempts have been made to provide health care to the people, who have remained largely on the periphery. However, no drastic policy measures have been taken toward the structural changes of the health care system. Understandably, structural changes in large organizations and bureaucracies are difficult to achieve and rarely come by. In addition, structural changes are economically expensive. More often than not bureaucracies do their best to avoid having to make structural changes. But in a poor developing country, such changes are necessary if social justice is to be achieved.

The major hindrances to the formulation of more effective health systems would appear to be the value systems of the elite groups and agencies and the structures these produce. Attempts to solve priority problems among the largest proportion of the population leave much to be desired. Existing health structures fly

103

in the face of available evidence on effective systems and strategies. In the conflict between political necessity and economic reality many problems have been avoided rather than solved. These problems do not disappear; they grow and magnify. It is the problems we have ignored, rather than those we have failed to conquer, that are constant difficulties. The challenge of modern health care practice is to design systems that are not only fair and just to all but efficient and effective.

If Kenyans of African extraction found the colonial health system unjust, they must also strive to create a system that is not disproportionately favorable to a few, as is the case in urban Kenya and especially among the "professionals." The African black elites, formerly "native elites," have inherited the formerly exclusive European and Asiatic tastes: hospitals, private clinics, and, inevitably, class distinctions. The professionalization currently pursued may not be in the best interest of the majority for very few will ever be able to afford the high professional fees. As George Bernard Shaw once said, "Every profession is a conspiracy against the public." Modifying that statement somewhat, Rene Dubos said that individualized health care, common among specialists, entrenches the status quo, which means that the control of those conditions which lead to individual community-wide problems is progressively less important except in rhetoric.[18] Political action is necessary to make relevant and viable socio-economic changes. Kenya's socio-economic system follows the free enterprise philosophy long established during the colonial days and now advanced to a very high degree. Within this development, ideology, democracy, and social justice are expected to thrive. One common index of these goals should be the distribution of social services among Kenyans. The performance of Kenya's politico-administrative institutions should be assessed in that context.

Expansion of the health services, if effective in providing preventive and basic curative care, will be a contribution toward socio-economic democratization. In a fundamental manner democracy must also include equitable accessibility to the basic needs of life, of which health is one. The question in this chapter is directed toward how far the existing system and its institutions can produce the expansion of health services necessary to bring health to the whole population.

NOTES

1. Medical Department, Kenya, *Annual Report* (Nairobi: Government Printer, 1927).
2. W. Rodney, *How Europe Underdeveloped Africa* (Washington: Howard University Press, 1974).
3. *Annual Report* (1927).
4. See Medical Department, Kenya, *Annual Reports* for 1949 and 1953.
5. E. Stainbrook, "Health and Disease and the Changing Social and Cultural Environment of Man." *American Journal of Public Health* 51 (1961): 1005.
6. A. Beck, *A History of the British Medical Administration of East Africa, 1900-1950* (Cambridge: Harvard University Press, 1970).
7. M. Malone, "The Rule of the Churches in the Health Services of Kenya: Twenty Years of Growth and Expansion. 1958-1978." Paper read at the *1st Annual Conference of Kenya Medical Research Institute*, Nairobi, 1980; C. W. Hartwig, "Church-related relations in Kenya: Health Issues." *Social Science Medicine* 13C (1979): 121.
8. Hartwig, "Church-related Relations."
9. Malone, "The Role of Churches."
10. Beck, *History*.
11. A. Beck, "History of Medicine and Health Services in Kenya (1900-1950)" in *Health and Disease in Kenya*, ed. L. C. Vogel et al. (Nairobi: EALB, 1974), pp. 44-58.
12. *Annual Report* (1949, 1953).
13. *Annual Report* (1949), p. 34.
14. R. Michels, *Political Parties* (New York: Free Press, 1962).
15. B. Abel-Smith, *Poverty, Development and Health Policy* (Geneva: World Health Organization, 1978); M. King, *Medical Care in Developing Countries* (Nairobi: Oxford University Press, 1966); O. Gish, *Planning for the Health*

Sector, the Tanzanian Experience (London: Croom Helm, 1975).

16. See Ministry of Finance and Economic Planning, Kenya, *Department Plans for 1964-1970, 1970-1974, 1974-1978, 1978-1983* (Nairobi: Government Printer, 1964, 1970, 1974, 1978); I. Illich, *Medical Nemesis* (New York: Pantheon Books, 1976); V. Djukanovich and E. P. Mach, *Alternative Approaches to Meeting Basic Health Needs in Developing Countries* (Geneva: World Health Organization, 1975); K. Newell, *Health by the People* (Geneva: World Health Organization, 1975).

17. F. M. Mburu, "Rhetoric Implementation Gap in Health Policy and Health Services Delivery in a Developing Country," *Social Science and Medicine* 13A (1979): 577.

18. R. Dubos, *Mirage of Health* (Garden City: Anchor Books, 1959).

6

COLONIAL RULE, INTERNATIONAL AGENCY AND HEALTH: THE EXPERIENCE OF GHANA

Patrick A. Twumasi

The Colonial Experience

A colonial system binds a colony by political and economic ties that promote the interests of the dominant country. The relationship depends on the opportunities which the resources of the colony offer, and on the power of the dominant society to exploit these resources.[1]

Ghana is the former British colony of the Gold Coast, but it is difficult to specify the exact beginning of its colonial experience. Historians claim that the first contact between Europeans and the people of the Gold Coast was in the fifteenth century by explorers searching for lucrative trade arrangements.[2] European explorers found the disease environment along the West Coast of Africa to be extremely dangerous. In particular they feared malaria and yellow fever. The Portuguese found the region so inhospitable that having arrived in the Gold Coast in 1471 they vacated their post in 1595 when they were challenged by the Dutch.[3] The British government formed the African Company of Merchants in 1750 partly to find adequate means to control or eradicate epidemic diseases in the West Coast. The government subsidized the company to the extent of £13,000 per annum. The company displaced the Dutch in 1821.[4] The death rate and morbidity figures were so high that two British governors existed at any one time so that one could be on sick leave. In 1899 Mary Kingsley wrote that the West Coast had a reputation for diseases.[5]

Attempts followed to improve health conditions. In the middle of the nineteenth century the British colonial administration decided to build hospitals in commercial and administrative centers. The few postal agencies were given anti-malaria drugs to distribute to government clerical officers, and to sell cheaply to local people. British medical officers were posted to the region; they were to develop a Gold Coast Medical Department and Services. Clinics were located in cities and principal towns where colonists engaged in commercial and mining activities. This was the beginning of an urban-centered health service. Modern curative medicine was formally institutionalized in the Gold Coast with the building of hospitals and dispensaries. The Basel Mission and the Catholic Mission introduced medical missionaries in rural centers "to penetrate into the heart of Africa to convert pagans to Christianity."[6] Their hospitals and clinics in rural Ghana today bear testimony to their sympathy with the poor and with rural people.

The colonial administration's medical policy recognized the importance of preventive health work. Preventive health measures were mainly intended to improve the health environment of government officials. Separate housing was developed to protect the health of expatriates. Top government officials, merchants and officials of mining companies were given bungalows. Modern water supply and the sanitary disposal of sewerage were concentrated in a few places. Later on, supporting domestic, clerical, and technical staff were also given medical coverage. They were medically screened and allowed to benefit from the new technology of modern medicine because they were carriers or possible carriers of infection. In other words, cultural isolation was found to be an ineffective preventive measure. It was gradually recognized that epidemic diseases could only be uprooted when the causative organism was located and neutralized. People, whether expatriates or locals, could not be isolated effectively in different localities.

Local people were recruited to start medical work in nursing, dispensaries and laboratories. Kisseih, a former chief nursing officer in the Ministry of Health, has noted that mission and colonial medical officers enlisted the help of male orderlies in 1878 "to bathe and to feed the sick, to dress wounds and to administer drugs to the local population under their medical supervision."[7] The first British colonial nursing sister arrived in the country at the same time.

The colonial health service had a rough beginning. Initial opposition seemed to come from the indigenous population. Traditional social structure and culture gave credence to social and spiritual theories of disease causation. Traditional cosmology seemed opposed to scientific conceptions of disease. The people failed to understand scientific explanation and experimentation in laboratories; these seemed irrelevant because immutable supernatural laws were the cause of illnesses. Traditional health practitioners monopolized the market for health care outside the family efforts at self-help.

In confronting the indigenous system, the British colonial administrators devised a method to neutralize the influence of the healers. A campaign of "enlightenment" was used to persuade city dwellers, the educated, and other opinion leaders that traditional healers were insincere and ignorant. The healers were consistently discredited in the popular media. Fearing prosecution, many healers returned to rural areas to practice in secrecy. The colonial administrator did not recognize the practice of traditional healing. If a person worked for the government, a mining company or in a commercial enterprise, he was expected to seek medical aid from the health service. Government medical officers were the only authorized people to issue an authentic health certificate to a worker or an official when he was found ill and was unable to attend work.

In their own way the missionaries also added their voice to "downgrade" the practice of traditional medicine. Their followers were encouraged to shun the healers. It was against Christian dogma to seek medical help from traditional healing. The healers were known as "fetish healers," "magical men," and "medicine men" who did not know the actual causes of disease.

Traditional healing was not entirely destroyed during the colonial period, but its image was tarnished and its evolution into modernity was halted. In the post-colonial period nationalists have rediscovered the place of traditional medicine in Ghanian society.[8] It is important for interdisciplinary research teams to study traditional medicine. At present a center for the analysis of traditional herbs has been instituted. Its work is to disentangle facts from beliefs about the efficacy of native herbs.

In a paradoxical way, in helping to fight diseases in the tropics, the modernization process introduced by the colonial administrators also helped to introduce new diseases and to spread infectious diseases quickly through the country. These were unintended social consequences of introducing social services. Because of an improved transportation system, it was much quicker and easier for people to move from place to place, and in many cases they carried their infections with them. Rural-urban migrants were effective agents in carrying diseases. Epidemics spread quicker than before. Hartwig and Patterson noted that government policies and the people's responses to them often created conditions favorable to the spread of diseases.[9] Drainage of land, the introduction of gutters and clearing sites for development projects created new niches for infectious organisms. As with much of the rest of the world in 1918, the Gold Coast experienced a nationwide epidemic of influenza. It reached many parts of the country and the damage was quite extensive. Today many old people still remember the influenza. Mark Delancey's essay on the German labor program in Cameroon is another excellent illustration of the effects of an improved transportation system.[10] He argued that European employers needed workers on large-scale plantations and other labor-extensive projects, and therefore encouraged large-scale population movements. The workers often lived in squalor. Migration and poor conditions in crowded cities contributed to the rapid spread of diseases. Sidney Kark and Guy Stuart discussed the rule of the returning migrants in carrying venereal diseases to the rural areas. Syphilis in northern Ghana was known as the "Kumasi Sickness."[11]

Thus, in the early part of the twentieth century the British colonial health administrators faced problems of how to control epidemic diseases, how to treat high fevers, how to prevent cross-infection, and how to immunize people against the deadly tropical diseases. In 1924 a medical complex was built in Accra to treat patients and to conduct research in tropical medicine. This was the Korle Bu Hospital complex, which is now the national center for training doctors. A British colonial governor, Sir Gordon Guggisberg, initiated and built the hospital during his tenure of office.

During the early decades, population increased dramatically. Health statistics show that in 1901 there were 1.9 million people in the area that today is Ghana, and that in 1911 there were 2.1 million people. In 1921 the census recorded 2.5 million people, and by 1931 numbers had increased to 3.5 million people. Death and disability rates among expatriate population improved after the discovery by Ross in 1898 of the mode of transmission of malaria (Table 1).[12]

Table 1

DEATH AND DISABILITY RATES AMONG EXPATRIATES
FOR THE YEARS 1923-24 AND 1933-34

Occupations	No. of people	Deaths	Death rate/ 1000	Invalids	Disability rates/100
1923-1924:					
Officials	994	10	10.1	32	32.2
Merchants	1425	11	7.7	25	17.5
Mining companies	527	2	3.8	28	53.1
Missionaries	97	1	10.3	2	20.6
Total	3043	24	7.9	87	28.6
1933-1934:					
Officials	847	3	3.5	42	49.0
Merchants	1359	6	4.4	13	9.6
Mining companies	682	8	11.7*	22	32.1
Missionaries	247	1	4.0	5	20.2
Total	3145	18	5.7	82	26.1

Source: *The Gold Coast Hand Book*, pp. 141. Crown Agents, Government Publications, London, 1937.

*More mines were opened and the hazards of finding new mining areas accounted for the increase in death rate among miners in 1933-1934 figures. The risk was great.

111

Collaborative Work of International Agencies

After World War II, it became increasingly clear that international health programs should be intensified. New media of communication and travel had given rise to rapid exchange of people and information among many parts of the world. The international community genuinely could be described by the slogan, "one world." The creation of the World Health Organization (WHO) acknowledged this fact. WHO held a conference in Ghana in 1954 at which experts discussed measures to be used in treating onchocerciasis.[13] The creation of the Volta Lake as a result of the country's industrialization programs had brought the disease to Ghana by creating a niche for the sand fly which acts as the vector. Consequently, research scientists directed their attention to the northern part of Ghana to embark upon a mass eradication and treatment program.

In the field of health education and population control, the Ford Foundation, the Population Council, and other multilateral agencies have given scholarships to train Ghanaian health personnel. In a paper entitled, "A philosophy of health work in the African region" WHO's Africa Regional Office notes that WHO spends some $2 million annually in awarding fellowships for African students to study abroad.[14] At the twenty-second World Health Assembly in 1970 the director general submitted a report which stated that in the African region "malaria remains the most important public health problem affecting as it does more than half the children under three years of age and virtually the whole population over that age, directly causing 10 percent of the deaths of children under five years of age."[15]

The colonial heritage left an urban-oriented health care system in the Gold Coast. Hospitals and clinics are located in cities. Doctors, nurses, and paramedical workers are interested primarily in curative practice. The few supporting services such as modern education, physical facilities (modern water supply, electricity and modern drainage system) are located in the cities and principal towns. With the exception of a few missionary hospitals and clinics, the rural areas are without modern health facilities. Most of the health professionals in the colonial civil service were expatriates; the approach of independence created a vacuum when many of them resigned.

112

The Nationalist Period

In 1957 the Gold Coast attained independence. The Nkrumah government inherited a good civil service administration, manpower, and a desire for ushering Ghana quickly into modern ways of life. Nkrumah's government decided to increase training for health workers and the facilities for practice. Many health centers were built during his administration (Table 2).

Table 2

HEALTH CENTERS IN OPERATION IN GHANA

Region	1957	1958	1959	1960	1961	1962	1963
Western	0	0	1	2	4	4	6
Central	0	1	1	2	2	2	2
Eastern	1	1	3	4	6	8	12
Volta	1	2	3	3	3	3	3
Ashanti	1	1	1	2	3	3	5
Brong Ahafo	2	2	2	4	4	7	7
Northern	3	3	3	3	3	4	4
Upper	2	2	2	2	2	2	2
Total	10	12	16	22	27	33	41

Source: See Ghana Government Publication. *The Health Services in Ghana*, p. 47. Ministry of Health, Accra, 1967.

In 1950, seven years before independence, there were 2800 students in the secondary schools. By 1964, seven years after independence, there were 28,100 students attending secondary schools. Many new schools and several colleges were built. New universities were instituted: the University of Science and Technology and the University of Cape Coast. The former was created initially to train middle calibre science and technology professionals. In 1964 the University of Science and Technology began training pharmacists and dispensary technicians. Also in 1964, the first medical school was opened at the facilities of the Korle Bu Hospital. It became part of the University of Ghana, the country's first university. Fifty medical students started their education at the university that year. Nursing training was intensi-

113

fied by building more colleges and by encouraging experienced Ghanaian nurses to study to become tutors and administrators by enrolling at the new Department of Post-Basic Nursing at the University of Ghana. In 1963 there were 904 doctors in the civil service (Table 3). From this number 78 percent were registered Ghanian doctors. There was one doctor to a population of 10,000 people.

Table 3

MEDICAL AND NURSING PERSONNEL
IN GOVERNMENT SERVICE

Personnel	1957	1958	1959	1960	1961	1962	1963
Doctors	330	342	346	586	726	879	904
Dentists	18	14	17	17	22	29	36
Midwives	616	691	789	900	1008	1104	1235
Nurses	800	986	1627	1848	2023	2191	2366
Pharmacists	312	311	326	298	329	342	355

Source: *Statistical Year Book*, p. 33. Central Bureau of Statistics, Accra, Ghana, 1963. Also see (8, p. 67).

In the immediate post-colonial period the curative as contrasted with preventive emphasis was still maintained. It was prestigious for the nationalist government to build more hospitals and clinics. Figures from the Ministry of Health show that in the seventies most money by far went into curative services (Table 4). Preventive services are not fashionable. It is expensive to build a sanitary system with modern water supplies, adequate drainage and sewerage systems. Although, in the long run, when its effect is felt by lowering preventable diseases, it becomes economic to undertake the expense.

The Ghanaian doctors who inherited the colonial structure maintained the Ghanaian colonial system. They were the new elite and stayed in the cities and the principal towns where supporting facilities were available, including good schools for their children and an elitist urban life suited to the "new colonials." The disease map of the country showed the prevalence of communicable and preventable diseases. The death rate figures were being reduced in

114

the urban areas but in the rural sector death among children and nursing mothers was still very high. Authorities attributed the high infant mortality to poor environmental sanitation, and to ignorance and superstition on the part of mothers.

Table 4

PERCENTAGE DISTRIBUTION OF HEALTH EXPENDITURE

Type of service	1973/74	1974/75	1975/76
Preventive	12.3	10.3	9.7
services	77.1	76.3	75.9
Curative services	0.2	0.4	0.5
Research activities	10.4	13.0	13.9
Administrative			
	100.0	100.0	100.0
Total			

Source: Ghana Government, Ministry of Health, *Health Planning Unit paper*, 1977.

Treating infectious and other diseases is a high priority in any developing country but the tendency to emphasize curative medicine at the expense of public health is a serious fault. While only 23 percent of the population lived in the urban areas, 76 percent of the doctors practiced there.[16] The figures for other medical and paramedical personnel are similar.

It is a standard assumption in Ghana that government workers who are sent to the rural areas are being punished by administrators. The professionals have effective power because of their prestige, scarcity, and social contacts with political decision makers to determine where to work. The rural areas are populated by people who have little or no comparable power and are unable to get sufficient amenities to meet their health needs. It is true that the urban population has been growing at a rapid pace and therefore logical to find that hospitals and their major health services concentrate in the urban areas. It is also reasonable to find that health professionals are attracted to urban areas because of the availability of supporting services and facilities.

The point we need to stress is that the limitation of resources strongly influences health planning. Modern health resources are expensive and often imported. Foreign exchange resources are scarce. If the present determinants for health planning continue in effect, then the urban-rural imbalance of the colonial structure will also remain.

Local Responses and Local Adaptation

For economic and practical reasons the colonial administrators developed modern health technology to protect their citizens against tropical diseases. Because the expatriate population was mainly located in the cities and large towns, an urban center health service was created. It would have been almost impossible to exploit the resources in the Gold Coast without taking measures to improve the health conditions in the country.

Research scientists, doctors, and paramedical personnel from many countries were recruited by international agencies in the fight against tropical diseases. This work gave new experiences to young scientists and health practitioners. As appropriately pointed out by Taylor, the principal motivation was self interest, but not selfishness.[17] The churches also joined in the fight against deadly diseases partly for altruistic reasons and partly because they wanted to convert local people to the Christian religion.

Today, health planners, university lecturers, and students challenge the existing health structure. Many of them come from the rural areas and wish to bargain effectively for their people. In Ghanaian society success is measured by how effective a person is in redistributing economic resources to his home district.

International agencies again have played an important role in directing the attention of the nationalist government to the rural people. Family planning ideas were introduced by an international agency, the Population Council. In 1970 the government outlined a national policy and asked local officials to coordinate activities in lowering the fertility rate. The majority of the people who have large families live in the rural areas. The death rate among children in rural areas also is high. From an ethical viewpoint family planning expresses the wish to improve the health needs of the rural folks.[18] The University of Ghana Medical School, in conjunction with the Ministry of Health, developed the Danfa Project to

116

train medical students in rural health practices and research.[19] In collaboration with the School of Public Health, University of California, Los Angeles, the Ghana Medical School assumed joint responsibility for the project. The Danfa Project contributed to research in rural health: it demonstrated the need for community health, for integration of family planning and health behavior; the need to tackle health needs from an interdisciplinary perspective; trained middle level health technicians, and instituted a training scheme to train traditional birth attendants.

Since Danfa, the Ghana Government and the World Health Organization have carried out another community health project in the Brong Ahafo region in Ghana. Its focus was to determine practical ways to reach rural communities with a comprehensive health scheme. The basic principle was to motivate local people in villages to share the responsibility in caring for their health and welfare. Health care must be accessible to the users and relevant to their needs. Also, it must integrate its activities with other developmental programs. In a recent study the Institute of Development Studies Health Group observed that "it [was] now accepted that in most countries of Africa, Asia, and Latin America, the government health services have failed to meet the needs of the rural masses. Too many children die of preventable illness."[20] This is true in Ghana also, although there is little agreement over what should be done.

Conclusion

What is taking place in Ghana is a combination of several major factors. First, there is an increasing awareness among the population that health care facilities, public health, the building of physical infrastructures and the education of the people are interrelated. Second, a perspective has been developed through modern education that the rulers are not just "governors" but are men and women who, being at the top of affairs, are expected to improve the health of the people. Modern education therefore has played an important role in helping to instigate the people to react to governmental health policies and programs. Third, in the districts and regional centers, a vocal group of modern councillors have emerged. In the village, voluntary associations, mainly welfare

117

and cooperative organizations, have sprung up to educate the people about their rights and obligations.

The central government has accepted the role of developing a primary health care system for the country. It is through this system that the vast majority of the rural people can receive primary health care. The National Health Planning Unit is responsible for seeing to the implementation of rural medical coverage.

> The unit has recommended the recruitment and training by the year 2000 of 22,000 community level primary health workers, who would be selected and supervised by village development committees and who would be involved in pregnancy management, first level medical care, environmental sanitation, health education and the mobilization of health related community projects.[21]

The success of its implementation is yet to be seen. It requires the availability of economic reserves, the use of intermediate technology, the retraining of professional health practitioners (in service education) and the decentralization of authority, so that at the village level the necessary feedback can be provided to monitor and to evaluate the system.

As we have noted, health systems have broad ranging ties with people's cosmology, their philosophical outlook, with their socio-economic structure and, indeed, their entire way of life. In this study it is at least clear that colonialism and international agencies were change agents. They have contributed to the development of modern health care in Ghana. But as an unintended social consequence of change, the functional equilibrium of the society had been affected. It is up to the national government to implement a health plan which fits into the overall societal networks. In tackling this challenge the government must recognize the changing needs of the people and the fact that in health care development there is an international interest and goodwill. Ghana owes much to the international community for its contribution to international health, but in the final analysis any evolving health care system, if it is to be adequately implemented to reach villages, must be designed locally to suit local needs.

NOTES

1. See the *Encyclopedia of the Social Sciences*, Vol. 3 (New York: Macmillan, 1937), pp. 651-53.
2. The *Gold Coast Handbook* (London: Crown Agents for the Colonies, 1937), p. 133; C. Hughes and J. M. Hunter, "Disease and Development in Africa," *Social Science and Medicine* 111 (1979): 443.
3. H. A. Wieschhoff, *Colonial Policies in Africa* (New York: Negro University Press, 1944); R. E. Dumett, "The Campaign Against Malaria and the Extension of Scientific Medical and Sanitary Services in British West Africa, 1899-1910," *African Historical Studies* 1 (1968): 17-36.
4. *Gold Coast Handbook* (1937), p. 10.
5. Mary Kingsley, *West Africa Studies* (New York: Macmillan, 1899).
6. Kingsley, *West Africa Studies*, p. 24.
7. Dorcia A. N. Kisseih, "Developments in Nursing in Ghana," *International Journal of Nursing Studies* 205 (1968); *Colonial Office Report on the Gold Coast* (London: Crown Agents, 1949), pp. 1-11.
8. Patrick A. Twumasi, *Medical Systems in Ghana: A Study in Medical Sociology* (Accra: Ghana Publishing, 1975); P. A. Twumasi, "A Sociological Perspective on the Problems of Adapting Modern Scientific Medicine to the Needs of a Developing Country," *Universitas* 3 (1974).
9. Gerald W. Hartwig, and K. David Patterson (eds.), *Disease in African History* (Durham: Duke University Press, 1978); L. David Patterson, "River Blindness in Northern Ghana 1900-1950," pp. 88, 153.
10. M. Delancey, "Health and Disease on the Plantations of Cameroon 1884-1939." In *Disease in African History*, ed. Gerald Hartwig and David Patterson, p. 153.

11. S. Kark, and G. Stuart (eds.), *A Practice of Social Medicine* (Edinburgh: Macmillan, 1960).

12. *The Gold Coast Handbook* (1937), p. 133.

13. WHO Expert Committee Second Report, *Simulium and Onchocerciasis in the Northern Territories of the Gold Coast* (Geneva: World Health Organization, 1956), p. 42.

14. World Health Organization, *A Philosophy of Health Work in the African Region*. Afro Technical Papers, No. 1. Regional Office for Africa (Brazzavelle: World Health Organization, 1970).

15. World Health Organization, *A Philosophy*, p. 113.

16. *Health Care, Health Services and the Rural Community*. A Report to the Government of Ghana, Vol. 1. IDS Health Group, Institute of Development Studies, University of Sussex, Brighton, Sussex, in collaboration with ISSER, University of Ghana, Legon, Ministry of Health and Department of Community Health, Korle Bu, Ghana.

17. Carl E. Taylor, "Changing Patterns in International Health: Motivation and Relationship," *American Public Health Journal* 9 (1971): 158.

18. Alfred K. Neuman, Frederick K. Wurapa, Irvin M. Lourie, and Samuel Ofosu Amaah, "Strategies for Strengthening Health Services Infrastructure: A Case Study in Ghana," *Social Science and Medicine* 130 (1979): 23-31.

19. Neuman, "Strategies," p. 129.

20. *Health Care*, p. 1.

21. See D. M. Warren, and Mary Ann Tregoning Sr., "Indigenous Healers and Primary Health Care in Ghana," *Medical Anthropology* Newsletter (1979): 11.

Part III: Contemporary Crisis and Contradictions

7

SOCIAL SCIENCE AND MEDICINE IN AFRICA

Isidore S. Ubot

Introduction

The direct involvement of social science and social scientists in medicine in the West (especially in the U.S.) started during the mid-1930s even though the relevance of psychology to medicine was recognized as far back as 1911.[1] By the 1950s sociologists in medical schools were engaged in the selection of students with the "right" attributes for medical training. Psychologists also were administering psychiatric tests to prospective students. Since then the numbers of behavioral scientists in American medical schools and schools of public health have increased tremendously over the years.[2]

This reported gain in the numerical strength of social scientists in American health care institutions in recent years is the result of both a recognition of behavioral components in diseases and a growing public disaffection with a strictly biomedical approach to health care. The recognition of the role of social and behavioral factors has been sided by the realization that beside morbidity and mortality caused by infectious and parasitic diseases, there are chronic disorders such as cancer, coronary heart disease, diabetes, and hypertension which are related to behavior and lifestyle. The inability of medicine to control these "new" problems has contributed to a general dissatisfaction with the predominant paradigm of medical practice which emphasizes cure and gives little weight to prevention. In an attempt to change the situation, a biopsychosocial (wholistic) model of medicine has been proposed. The primary health care (PHC) approach which takes into account social, environmental, and psychological factors in health and illness has been accepted, at least in principle, in many parts of the world.[3]

Medical sociologists, anthropologists, psychologists, and physicians with social science biases have contributed significantly to the emergence of this new world view. In one of the more famous critiques of medicine John and Sonja McKinley have clearly demonstrated the role of social factors in disease and illness. From analysis of available data on mortality from ten infectious diseases in the U.S. they made a convincing case for the position that "the introduction of specific medical measures and/or the expansion of medical services are generally not responsible for most of the modern decline in mortality".[4]

In "Determinants of Health," McKeown has criticized what he calls "the engineering approach to medicine" and has attributed the modern decline in mortality not to developments in medicine but to socio-economic factors. Using data from eighteenth and nineteenth century England and Wales he concluded that

> the death rate from infectious diseases fell because an increase in food supplies led to better nutrition. From the second half of the nineteenth century this advance was strongly supported by improved hygiene and safer food and water, which reduced exposure to infection. With the exception of smallpox vaccination, which played a small part in the total decline of mortality, medical procedures such as immunization and therapy had little impact on human health until the twentieth century.[5]

While recognizing that today's problems in the West are with non-communicable diseases with significant behavioral components (cancer, heart disease, cerebrovascular disease), McKeown still warns against an individually-based, curative health care:

> The role of individual medical care in preventing sickness and premature death is secondary to that of other influences; yet society's investment in health care is based on the premise that it is the major deter-

124

minant. It is assumed that we are ill and made well, but it is nearer the truth that we are well and made ill.[6]

The view of health expressed in these statements reflects the position taken in earlier works by McKeown which asserts that disease and health are socially determined and that medicine does not keep us well.[7]

Social Science and Medicine in Africa

The emphasis on prevention which these views imply has implications particularly to health and illness in Africa. Though a new pattern of disorders is emerging especially among urban elites, the old scourges of mankind—malaria, diarrhoea, typhoid, cholera, and yellow fever—still remain the major causes of death in Africa.[8] With these diseases on the rampage and with slow progress in the development of relevant sectors, the state of health of Africans has remained precarious. In many countries, for example Nigeria and Malawi, the infant mortality rate is more than 100 per 1000 live births; life expectancy is below or slightly above fifty years; the quality and quantity of food consumed are grossly inadequate; and the ratio of health manpower to population is at an unsatisfactory level.[9] In the period between 1981 and 1985, economic development (as can be judged from per capita GNP) has, at best, stagnated in many African countries (Table 1). Considering the prevalence of the old problems of drought, wars, dependency, and mismanagement of available resources, the health projections for the year 2000 cannot but show a bleak future especially since pragmatic policies may not be formulated and/or implemented in the health sector in the near future.

In response to the health problems in Africa and in order to bring about a desired (healthful) future, social scientists have contributed in different ways to health development in the continent. For many years they have been engaged in studies which have sought to highlight the relationship of economic, cultural, political, and social psychological factors to health. Running through many of the studies is the relationship between health and political economy. The implication of this argument is that health policy cannot be divorced from the power

Table 1
HEALTH AND RELATED DATA FOR
SELECTED AFRICAN COUNTRIES

Countries	Population (millions)		GNP ($)[1]		Life Expectancy (years)	
	1981	1985	1981	1985	1981	1985
Benin	3.6	4.0	320	260	50	49
Congo, P.R.	1.7	1.9	1110	1110	60	58
Cote d'Ivorie	8.5	10.1	1200	660	47	53
Ethiopia	3.2	42.3	140	110	46	45
Ghana	11.8	12.7	400	380	54	53
Kenya	17.4	20.4	420	290	56	54
Liberia	1.9	2.2	520	470	54	50
Malawi	6.2	7.0	200	160	44	45
Nigeria	87.6	94.7	870	800	49	50
Senegal	5.9	6.6	430	370	44	47
Tanzania	19.1	22.2	280	290	52	52
Togo	2.7	3.0	380	230	48	51
Zaire	29.8	30.6	210	170	50	51
Zambia	5.8	6.7	600	390	51	52

Countries	Total Fertility Rate[2]		Infant Mortality Rate[3]		Child Death Rate	
	1981	1985	1981	1985	1981	1985
Benin	6.5	6.5	152	115	33	19
Congo, P.R.	6.0	6.3	127	77	26	7
Cote d'Ivorie	6.8	6.5	125	105	25	15
Ethiopia	6.5	6.2	145	168	31	38
Ghana	7.0	6.4	101	94	19	11
Kenya	8.0	7.8	85	91	15	16
Liberia	6.9	6.9	152	127	33	23
Malawi	7.8	7.6	169	156	38	35
Nigeria	6.9	6.9	133	109	28	21
Senegal	6.5	6.7	145	137	31	27
Tanzania	6.5	7.0	101	110	19	22
Togo	6.5	6.5	107	97	20	12
Zaire	6.3	6.1	110	102	21	20
Zambia	6.9	6.8	104	84	20	15

Countries	Population/ Physician 1981	1985	Urban Population (%) 1981	1985	Daily Calorie Supply/Capita[4] 1981	1985
Benin	12,390	17,000	15	35	2292	2173
Congo, P.R.	14,210	-	46	40	2277	2549
Cote d'Ivorie	19,080	-	41	45	2746	2505
Ethiopia	70,190	88,120	14	15	1735	1681
Ghana	13,670	7,250	37	32	1964	1747
Kenya	12,820	10,140	15	20	2078	2151
Liberia	12,400	9,400	34	37	2390	2311
Malawi	46,900	53,000	10	-	2095	2448
Nigeria	44,230	12,000	21	30	2595	2038
Senegal	21,100	14,200	34	36	2406	2342
Tanzania	21,700	-	12	14	2051	2335
Togo	23,200	21,200	21	23	2101	2236
Zaire	35,100	-	36	39	2180	2154
Zambia	11,400	7,800	44	48	2051	2137

Sources: World Bank, World Development Report (1983 and 1987 Editions). New York: Oxford University Press.

Notes: [1]Twelve of the fourteen countries recorded declines in per capita income between 1981 and 1985.

[2]This is the average number of children per woman living through her childbearing lifetime of 15-49 years. The rate is based on actual frequency of childbearing among women in that age group in a particular year.

[3]The number of infants below 1 year of age who die in one year per one thousand born live.

[4]Estimated per capita calories requires for normal daily activity is about 2500-3000. Less is required for sedentary life.

structure of any society and the nature of its economic relations.[10] Consequently the state of health of Africans can only be understood through analysis of their colonial past and present capitalistic structures.[11]

Ityavyar traced the origin of the overemphasis on tertiary (curative) care in Africa to Christian medical missions.[12] The major preoccupation of colonial health planners, he argues, was the development of curative centers in African cities and towns. In this era hospitals were built to treat infectious diseases like smallpox and malaria and catered to the health needs of Europeans, colonial bureaucrats, and a few well-placed Africans. Since this calibre of people generally lived in towns, the hospitals were built in urban areas.

This trend has continued to the present. First of all, health budgets have remained top-heavy, with allocations to the tertiary sector—building of hospitals, purchase of equipment, training and remuneration of high-level manpower. Preventive activities generally receive scant attention. Second, the distribution of available manpower and siting of hospitals and other facilities favor urban centers to the neglect of rural communities where most of the people live. In Nigeria, for example, with a rural population of up to 70 percent, about two-thirds of physicians live and work in towns.[13] An analysis of physician distribution by state has also shown an urban bias.[14] This bias is certainly not the result of shortage of manpower because even in countries where there is a surplus of physicians, maldistribution has remained an unfortunate phenomenon.[15]

The bias toward curative care is also reflected in the profile of specialty training in Nigeria. Of all the specialists trained between 1976 and 1985 in the country, less than 5 percent (9 out of 189) specialized in public health. Internal medicine, obstetrics and gynecology, surgery, pediatrics and pathology (in that order) were the most popular fields.[16] The limitations of an over-emphasis on urban-based curative care are many: planning tends to be centrally based; wastage of available resources is rampant; resource allocation is generally inadequate; and the delivery of care failed to reach those most in need. Moreover, the training of physicians for tertiary care requires the services of highly trained experts who are often in short supply. This problem has been bitterly felt in Nigeria where medical residents and consultants have left "centers of excellence" to more financially and professionally rewarding posts in the Gulf states. In Zambia's only medical school the shortage of lecturers is a palpable problem. Recently the president of the Medical Students' Association in the school decried the prospect of graduating "half-baked doctors".[17] Zambia is certainly not alone in this respect.

Because of the central role of appropriate manpower in health development, this area has received serious attention from social scientists. The focus here has been on the training of a new calibre of health care personnel. The emphasis is on rural based health manpower. According to Abba et al:

> Such manpower would be drawn from among the villagers themselves and would go back to live as part of the villager's division of responsibilities the way herbalists, traditional psychiatrists and traditional midwives have existed and worked within the rural community.[18]

The Chinese model of "barefoot doctors" has shown this to be an effective way of providing health care to the people. It has also been demonstrated that the type of manpower implied in this model is more in tune with the needs and feelings of rural dwellers and may influence the pattern of utilization of community health facilities.[19]

The underutilization of available health facilities has also been addressed in a systematic way by social scientists. The distrust with which rural people view health facilities seems to be one of the reasons for the underutilization of these facilities. Several other factors come into play. Okafor has shown that utilization is related to accessibility which in turn is related to other indices of socio-economic development.[20] Onucha found that underutilization is the result of faith in native doctors and midwives.[21] Other factors such as distance, time spent, cost and availability of drugs have been associated with the refusal to use available health facilities.[22]

These studies on different aspects of health in Africa are contributions by social scientists to the adoption of an effective framework for health development in the continent. The study to be reported below is a survey of activities and problems of social scientists directly involved in one health sector activity of training future physicians. Evidence from the U.S. has shown that though there has been a tremendous increase in absolute numbers of social scientists in medical institutions, the role of social science in medicine has remained a limited one. Social scientists in these institutions have complained of isolation from the mainstream of their disciplines, lack of appreciation of their contributions, and status inequality with their medically trained colleagues.[23] The necessity of an effective participation of African social scientists in all spheres of health development has been commented upon by both Ebigbo and Osuntokun.[24] What, then, is the extent of involvement of social science in African medical education and health care and how are the social scientists faring in their roles? A study was conducted to find this out.

Method

First, a list of social scientists was requested from the provosts and deans of colleges and faculties of medicine of twelve federal universities in Nigeria during the 1985-1986 session. Social scientists were specified as anthropologists, economists, political scientists, psychologists, and sociologists holding full-time appointments in the university and/or directly involved in the training of students and delivery of health care. A standard form was prepared and used to gather this information.

The questionnaires were sent by mail to the social scientists on the lists. They were provided with stamped, self-addressed envelopes for return of the questionnaires. Reminders were sent to those who did not respond within a specified period of time. Some questionnaires were collected by hand during visits to selected schools.

The questionnaire contained structured and open-ended questions. The instrument had three sections concerning demographic information, academic training, past and present employment; information on research, teaching and clinical activities; and professional problems and their opinions on health development in Nigeria. The questionnaire was constructed on the basis of information in the literature, discussions with social scientists, and the author's past experience as a social scientist in a college of medicine.

130

Results

The first objective of the study, as stated earlier, was to determine the number of social scientists engaged in medical education and health care in teaching hospitals. Information from the twelve schools showed a total of nineteen social scientists. All but two schools had at least one social scientist on the medical faculty. One school had four, another had three, four schools had two each, and another four schools had one each. The total of nineteen was made up of ten psychologists, eight sociologists, and one anthropologist. No school of medicine had an economist or political scientist on its faculty.

Analysis of departmental affiliations showed that the lone anthropologist, three psychologists, and four sociologists worked in departments of community health/social medicine, and six psychologists and one sociologist in departments of psychiatry/mental health. The rest (one psychologist and three sociologists) worked in other units, such as child health and psychological medicine. Seventy-five percent of them held doctorate degrees in their disciplines; some were registered for the Ph.D. programs in their institutions. The two predominant groups of social scientists were psychologists and sociologists. Both groups spent most time teaching, 33.75 percent and 38 percent respectively (Table 2). While sociologists spent an almost equivalent amount of time (35 percent) in research, psychologists spent the next higher amount of their time (25 percent) in clinical work. The difference in the time spent in clinical work between psychologists and sociologists (25 percent vs. 11 percent) reflects the fact that most of the psychologists (6) and only one sociologist worked in the departments of psychiatry/mental health.

Types of problems experienced. In order to determine the problems experienced by the social scientists in their work, a one variable chi-square (goodness-of-fit) test was conducted on the data on problems (Table 3). The analysis showed a significant chi-square ($X^2 = 5.33$, $p < .05$) on only one problem, that is perceived status inequality with medical colleagues.[25] There was a widespread though not statistically significant feeling that the administration showed a lack of interest in the work of social scientists. Students, on the other hand, were thought to show interest.

Table 2

MEAN PERCENT OF TIME SPENT IN DIFFERENT ACTIVITIES
BY PSYCHOLOGISTS AND SOCIOLOGISTS

Activity	Psychologists (n=6)	Sociologists (n=8)
Teaching	33.75	38.0
Basic Research	5.0	21.0
Applied Research	13.75	14.0
Clinical Work/health Care delivery	25.0	11.0
Administration	5.5	8.2
Consulting	17.0	7.8
Total	100.0	100.0

Table 3

ANALYSIS OF TYPES OF PROBLEMS EXPERIENCED BY
SOCIAL SCIENTISTS IN MEDICAL SCHOOLS

	Yes	No
1. Students' lack of interest in subject	4	8
2. Heavy teaching load	5	6
3. Too much clinical work	5	5
4. Status inequality with medical colleagues	10	2*
5. Administration's lack of interest in subject	6	2

*P < .05

The perceived need for social scientists in medical schools.
On why they thought their services were needed in medical
schools, most respondents agreed with the statements regarding
the motivations of the medical school administrators in hiring
them. Analyses of responses with the one-variable chi-square test
showed significant differences on items dealing with training in
patient/physician relations ($X^2 = 7.36$, $p < .01$). These and the

high rates of agreement with three other items in the list indicate that social scientists in medical schools believe strongly that their services are needed for genuine reasons. As shown earlier, this does not necessarily mean much interest in their work by medical school administrators.

Why the medical school? All except two of the social scientists in the sample stated that they could also have worked in the traditional departments of their disciplines within the university (anthropology, psychology, sociology). Why then did they choose the medical school as their primary place of employment? The reasons given were greater opportunity for research in the medical school (9), better pay (2), better opportunity for clinical work (2), and accessibility to other health professionals (1). Two respondents stated that positions were not available elsewhere.[26]

Courses of Instruction. The social scientists in this sample (n = 12) were asked to list the titles of the courses they were teaching. Courses listed included the following: medical ecology, medical psychology, medical sociology, introductory psychology, psychology and medicine, behavioral sciences, special topics in mental health, social epidemiology, socio-cultural factors in health and illness, demography, primary health care, and statistics. A look at selected catalogs of medical schools showed that most of these courses were listed for departments of community health and psychiatry. Credit load for each of the courses was one in most cases and rarely more than two hence the time spent on them was minimal. Generally the courses were taught in the preclinical years. The contact of social scientists with students in the clinical years was during field work (posting) in community health and psychiatry.

Additional findings. The opinion of respondents was sought on some health development issues. Many strongly agreed that contemporary health problems in Nigeria included not only infectious diseases but problems with major behavioral components (such as substance abuse, mental illness, and traffic accidents). Another finding showed a strong belief in the relevance of non-

133

physician manpower (including traditional practitioners) in African health development.

Discussion

The findings of this survey cannot be compared to earlier work on the involvement of social science in African medicine since none exists. Going by the review of contributions of social science and the results of the study, it seems clear that even though social scientists have made commendable analytical contributions to health their participation in the training of future health personnel is inadequate. One reason for this may be the dearth of social scientists with requisite qualifications and training to participate effectively in this health sector activity. After all there is a general scarcity of staff in many areas of medical education in Nigeria as in other African countries. Another reason is that even when qualified social scientists seek employment in colleges of medicine, administrators may refuse to hire them because of a fundamental lack of understanding of the role of social science in medicine.

It is true, of course, that the absolute increase in the number of social scientists in health institutions may not necessarily change the direction of Western medicine's engineering approach to health care. The American example is instructive in this regard. In spite of the impressive increases in the number of social scientists in medical schools in recent years, there remains a basic problem of integration of social science and biomedicine.[27]

Kleinman blames the marginality of social science in American medicine on several factors.[28] Within medicine there is the problem of an inherent bias toward the biomedical paradigm, a general bias against social scientists, inadequate exposure to social science courses in the premedical years, and differences in value hierarchies or "paradigms of practice" which make medical educators, researchers, and practitioners uncomfortable with social science. Within social science there are problems related to inadequate understanding of medicine, negative stereotypes of medicine and medical practitioners, and an unfavorable reward system in medical settings. Commenting on the situation in Australia, Kamien and Sanson-Fisher agree with Kleinman that the problem lies both in medicine's seemingly intractable biotechnological orientation and the shortcomings of the social science approach to medicine.[29]

Since medicine in African countries generally mimics Western medicine in its biotechnological emphasis, it is no surprise then that in medical schools social scientists often feel neglected and on the periphery of activities. Though not clearly articulated in the sample studied, some may even feel that they are used to "perform symbolic functions that essentially serve to legitimate the traditional structure and autonomous status of the medical profession."[30] In other words they may feel as if employed to work as hand maidens of biomedicine.

The feeling among social scientists in the sample studies that their role in medical education may not be taken seriously by administrators is supported by two observations. First, is the short shrift given to courses with social science content in the curriculum. Certainly, social scientists teach many courses as shown from the findings of this survey, but many of these are one credit courses. This means that contact hours with students are minimal and exposure to social science principles and their application to medical practice grossly inadequate. As if to tell students not to take their little time with the social sciences seriously, one Nigerian medical school, in a recent publication, informed students that "anatomy, biochemistry, physiology, and neuroscience are statutory [courses]. . . . The course in human psychology and medical sociology is given in the second semester by the departments of psychiatry and community health. There is no statutory examination in this subject." Probably because of the fear that students may not take the trouble of attending lectures in this course they are further informed that marks from evaluation of performance in the course are used in continuous assessment of students in the respective departments. With this attitude of medical school administrators who more often than not are ideologically committed to the hubris of biomedicine, it is no surprise that medical students taken community health courses in preclinical years and the clinical clerkshop less seriously than "real" medical courses.

The second issue of concern to social scientists in medical establishments is their inequality with physician members of faculty. In many African medical schools a non-physician, no matter his or her academic rank, cannot be the substantive head of a clinical department (including community health and psychiatry) even though he or she may be engaged in clinical activities; may not be paid clinical supplementation for his or her clinical work; and cannot be elected dean or provost of the school or college of medicine. The complaint of inequality expressed in this survey is therefore not surprising. In fact, one respondent inserted the comment that judging from his academic productivity he would have had a higher rank if he was a physician. Another (a clinical psychologist) blamed psychiatrists in his department for undermining his practice and rejecting equality.

The problems experienced by social scientists in medical establishments do not diminish their essential role in medicine and health. The problems only highlight the guild interests of medicine as a profession determined to protect its power. A total embrace of social scientists and the social science paradigm in medicine would imply a loss of some power to strangers. A ready acceptance of prevention as the focus of health care instead of technologically sophisticated treatments would mean a different definition is established and simple, preventive medicine would take the definition out of elite control.

As stated earlier in the introductory section of this chapter, health and disease are socially determined. Medicine's preoccupation with technological devices is antithetical to public health especially in Africa where easily preventable infectious and parasitic diseases and malnutrition are the major causes of morbidity and mortality. In line with the works of McKeown, McKinlay and McKinlay, and Navarro, an ineluctable truth has emerged: most of the disorders afflicting Africans are related to food and environmental sanitation, and most of the time, these disorders are found in rural areas among women and children.[31] The tragedy is that the deaths and illnesses can easily be prevented but are not. What is needed by African medical establishments and government is a new conception of health and policies which recognize the social nature of disease.

Conclusion

The survey reported in this chapter was conducted in Nigeria with a sample of twelve social scientists from a total reported number of nineteen. Even though this was a study of the situation in a single African country its relevance to the rest of the continent cannot be denied. The pattern of problems and stage of development of much of subsaharan Africa are very much alike (Table 1). Most Africans live in rural areas or in urban squalor and are confronted daily with hunger and disease. The limitations of traditional Western medical care can be found in all African countries and, indeed, are worldwide. The ongoing debate on the training of a new breed of doctors in the U.S. and the rest of the world is a sign of the crisis in Western medicine.[32]

It is becoming an increasingly acceptable idea that health cannot be divorced from political economic considerations and that prevention, not cure, is the way to achieve health for all.[33] Health policies aimed at eliminating the old and persistent problems or controlling the new ones demand the input of those trained in human behavior, culture, and society. Social scientists have already shown their ability to contribute through succinct analyses of the problems inherent in our health care system and effective participation in health care delivery.[34]

Yet, as this study has revealed, there are problems for the social scientist in his or her role as educator and practitioner. To overcome these problems different inputs are called for. For effective involvement in the training of a new breed of physicians, social scientists in medical schools need the support of medical school administrators and the medical establishment. Support for and understanding of the relevance of social science in health care activities can be shown through changing those policies which tend to perpetuate inequalities in the reward system thus inhibiting the progress of social scientists in medical establishments. To aid in this, social scientists themselves must be clear about the content and extent of their professional participation, and their self-identities as anthropologists, sociologists, economists, or psychologists.

In the second role of practitioner, concerted activism is called for at both individual and professional group levels. There is an ongoing need for the sensitization of policy makers to the concept of health for all and the interrelationship of health and economic development. This can be achieved through participation in debates on policy formulation and implementation and education of citizens on their right to health.[35]

A third role of social science in health development is in the area of research. The importance of objective data on African health cannot be overstressed. There are vast uncharted areas of research on culture and illness, health beliefs and practices, accident prevention, the behavior of health care providers, traditional health care, substance abuse, and so forth which call for more extensive interdisciplinary work by African social and medical scientists with professional interest in health development.

In conclusion, it is important to note that because this is a pioneer study in Africa further work is necessary. Also because of the small size of the sample (though constituting 63 percent of the population of social scientists) some of the findings need to be taken cautiously. Further work in the area will benefit from the inclusion of the views and reactions of medical school administrator and physicians concerning the role of social science and medicine in Africa.

Acknowledgement

This work was supported by Grant No. FRGC/1984-85/010 of the Faculty of Social Sciences, University of Jos. I thank Dennis Ityavyar and two anonymous reviewers for their comments on an earlier draft of this chapter.

NOTES

1. J. D. Matarazzo, "Behavioural Health's Challenge to Academic, Scientific and Professional Psychology," *American Psychologist* 37 (1982): 949-54.
2. R. L. Buck, "Behavioural Scientists in Schools of Medicine," *Journal of Health and Human Behaviour* 2 (1961): 59-64; J. Stokes, B. J. Strand, and C. Jaffe, "Distribution of Behavioural Science Faculty in United States Medical Schools 1968-69 and 1978-79," *Social Science and Medicine* 18 (1984): 753-56.
3. G. L. Engel, "The Need for a New Medical Model: A Challenge for Biomedicine," *Science* 196 (1977): 129-36; World Health Organization, *Primary Health Care* (Geneva: World Health Organization, 1978).
4. J. B. McKinley and S. M. McKinley, "Medical Measures and the Decline of Mortality," in *The Sociology of Health and Illness: Critical Perspectives*, ed. P. Conrad and R. Kern (New York: St. Martins, 1981), p. 13.
5. T. McKeown, "Determinants of Health," *Human Nature* 1/4 (1978): 60-67. Reference on pp. 64-65.
6. McKeown, "Determinants," p. 66.
7. T. McKeown, *The Role of Medicine: Dream, Mirage or Nemesis?* (Nuffield Provincial Hospitals Trust, 1976); T. McKeown, *The Modern Rise of Population* (New York: Academic Press, 1977).
8. B. O.Osuntokun, "Behaviour and Health," in *Psychology and Society*, ed. E. Wilson (Ile-Ife: Nigerian Psychological Association, 1986); B. O. Osuntokun, *The Health of the Public Servant and the Nation's Destiny*, Distinguished Lecture Series No. 3 (Kuru, Nigeria: National Institute for Policy and Strategic Studies, 1987); D. Ityavyar, "Aids Hysteria in Nigeria: A Strategy for Social Defence," paper presented at the Fourth Annual General Assembly of the

Social Science Council of Nigeria, ABU, Zaria, 1-3 June 1987; S. O. Alubo, "The 1986 Yellow Fever Epidemic in Nigeria: A Materialist Analysis," unpublished manuscript (Jos, University of Jos, 1987); Federal Office of Statistics, *Annual Abstract of Statistics* (Lagos: Federal Office of Statistics, 1985).

9. World Bank, *World Development Report* (New York: Oxford University Press, 1987).
10. V. Navarro, *Medicine Under Capitalism* (New York: Neal Watson, 1976); L. Doyal, *The Political Economy of Health* (London: Pluto Press, 1979).
11. S. O. Alubo, "Underdevelopment and the Health Care Crisis in Nigeria," *Medical Anthropology* 9/4 (1985): 319-35; O. Oculi, "Health and Imperialism," in *Health Problems in Rural and Urban Africa: A Nigerian Political Economy of Health Science*, ed. O. Oculi (Zaria: Ahmadu Bello University, 1981); O. F. Onoge, "Capitalism and Public Health: A Neglected Theme in the Medical Anthropology of Africa," in *Topias and Utopias in Health*, ed. S. R. Ingman and A. E. Thomas (The Hague: Mouton, 1975).
12. D.A. Ityavyar, "Background to the Development of Health Services in Nigeria," *Social Science and Medicine* 24/8 (1987): 487-99.
13. O.O. Akinkugbe, "A Third World Perspective," *World Health Forum* (April 1987): 24-25.
14. Oculi, "Health and Imperialism."
15. Z. Bankowski, "A Wasteful Mockery," *World Health Forum* (April 1987): 3-4.
16. Akinkugbe, "Third World Perspective."
17. Africa Health, "Prospect of 'Half-baked Doctors' in Zambia," *Africa Health* 9/3 (1987): 4.
18. A. Abba et al., *The Nigerian Economic Crisis: Causes and Solutions* (Zaria: Academic Staff Union of Universities of Nigeria, 1985), p. 138.
19. I. N. Egwu and I. S. Obot, "Nigerian Health Care: Reaching Out to the People," *The Health Service Journal* 97 (1987): 338.
20. F. C. Okafor, "Accessibility to General Hospitals in Rural Bendel State, Nigeria," *Social Science and Medicine* 18/8 (1984): 661-66.

21. G. B. I. Onucha, "Factors Responsible for Under-utilization of Available Health Services by the Rural People in Nigeria," *The Last African Medical Journal* 58/ii (1981): 859-66.

22. W. Gesler, "Illness and Health Practitioner Use in Calabar, Nigeria," *Social Science and Medicine* 13/D (1979): 23-30.

23. R. G. Nathan, G. Lubin, J. D. Matarazzo, and G. W. Persely, "Psychologists in Schools of Medicine, 1955, 1964, 1977," *American Psychologist* 34 (1979): 622-27.

24. P. E. Ebigbo, "The Psychologist Among Doctors: The UNTH Experience," in *Psychological Strategies for National Development*, ed. E. Okpara (Enugu: Nigerian Psychological Association, 1985); Osuntokun," Behaviour and Health."

25. It is important to note that because of the small size of the sample used in this study tests of significance must be treated with caution. Even though the significant findings reflect the pattern of responses, the strength of inference is diminished by the sample size.

26. The numbers add up to more than twelve because respondents could tick more than one item.

27. Buck, "Behavioural Scientists"; Stokes, Strand, and Jaffe, "Distribution of Behavioural Science Faculty."

28. A. Kleinman, "Some Uses and Misuses of the Social Sciences in Medicine," in *Metatheory in Social Science*, ed. D. W. Fiske and R. A. Sweder (Chicago: University of Chicago Press, 1986).

29. M. Kamien, "Commentary: Behavioural Science Is Not Spoken Here—Where Are the Interpreters?" *Community Health Studies* 8 (1983): 223-28; R. Sanson-Fisher, "Commentary: Behavioural Science and its Relation to Medicine—A Need for Positive Action," *Community Health Studies* 3 (1985): 275-83.

30. E. Riska, and P. Vinten-Johansen, "The Involvement of the Behavioural Sciences in American Medicine: A Historical Perspective," *International Journal of Health Services* 11 (1981): 583-96.

31. McKeown, *Role of Medicine*; McKeown, *Modern Rise of Population*; McKinley and McKinley, "Medical Measures"; Navarro, *Medicine Under Capitalism*; V. Navarro, "A Critique of the Ideological and Political Positions of the Willy Brandt

Report and the WHO Alma Ata Declaration," *Social Science and Medicine* 18 (1984): 467-74;

32. D. Bok, *The President's Report 1982-1983* (Cambridge: Harvard University, 1984); World Health Organization, "Wanted: A New Breed of Doctors," *World Health Forum* 6 (1985): 291-309.
33. Navarro, *Medicine Under Capitalism*; Navarro, "A Critique"; World Health Organization, *Primary Health Care*.
34. Ebigbo, "Psychologists Among Doctors."
35. J. S. Obot, "Social Science and Health for All (HFA)," paper presented at the Fourth Annual General Assembly of Bello University, Zaria, 1-3 June 1987.

8

THE UNDERDEVELOPMENT OF TRADITIONAL MEDICINE IN AFRICA

U. A. Igun

The relationship between traditional African and Western medicine has been studied from various perspectives and with varying aims. Studies of this relationship range from a hostile and nonchalant attitude towards traditional medicine at one extreme to a vigorous defensive attitude towards traditional medicine at the other. Those who condemn traditional medicine base their arguments on the assumed superiority of Western medicine and the reported non-scientific nature of traditional medicine. These studies go on to detail what they see as the dangers involved in utilizing traditional medicine. For example, they point at adverse side effects of the unproven and unprocessed herbs it uses and to misdiagnosis. The defenders of traditional medicine base their defence largely on the efficacy of many traditional medical practices. They also question the assumption of the unscientific nature of traditional medicine.[1]

The aim of this chapter is not to evaluate these claims specifically but to show why African traditional medicine has such low status in official thinking and why it has received very little positive attention. In other words, we shall try to show why it is an underdeveloped system. Further, we shall suggest ways of creating circumstances within which it could be developed and its potentials realized.

Traditional and Western Medicine and the Issue of Science

It has been argued by those who claim that Western medicine is superior to traditional African medicine, that traditional medicine is unscientific. Bonsi has argued convincingly that this claim is both arrogant and misleading. Following Dingwall, he points out that traditional thought is as interested in natural causes as Western science and that there is no clear difference between scientific and other forms of knowledge. Moreover, there is sufficient evidence to show that most of the postulates of traditional thought actually grasp reality.[2]

Horton's classic work has shown that there is no fundamental difference between Western scientific thought and African traditional thought.[3] What difference there is is merely the idiom in which thought is expressed which itself is a product of the socio-cultural and physical environment and technological level of society. Janzen, too, has argued that rationality is not synonymous with modern experimental science.[4] He pointed out that although Western medicine claims to be scientific, it is neither more nor less rational than the Kongo healing tradition which reasons that plants should be combined according to their origin from the village and the forest, or that an illness which does not respond to medications or manipulative therapy is likely to be caused by conflict, tension, or hostility in human interaction. Advocates may be attached dogmatically to their own system, each convinced his is rational or true. The following amusing exchange between David Livingstone (M.D.) and a Mbundu rainmaker reported by Janzen puts the case of the protagonists very well:

Medical Doctor: Hail, friend! How very many medicines you have about you this morning; why, you have every medicine in the country here.

Rain Doctor: Very true my friend; and I ought; for the whole country needs the rain which I am making.

M.D.:   So you really believe that you can command the clouds? I think that can be done by God alone.

R.D.:   We both believe the very same thing. It is God that makes the rain, but I pray to him by means of these medicines, and

144

the rain coming of course it is then mine. It was I who made it for the Bakwaine for many years, when they were at Shokuane; through my wisdom, too, their women became fat and shining. Ask them; they will tell you the same as I do.

M.D.: But we are distinctly told in the parting words of our Saviour that we can pray to God acceptably in his name alone, and not by means of medicines.

R.D. : Truly, but God told us differently. He made black men first and did not love us as he did the white man. He made you beautiful, and gave you clothing, and guns, and gunpowder, and horses, and wagons, and many other things about which we know nothing. But towards us he had no heart. He gave us nothing except the assagai, and cattle, and rainmaking; and he did not give us hearts like yours. We never love each other. Other tribes place medicines about our country to prevent the rain, so that we may be dispersed by hunger, and flee to them, and augment their power. We must dissolve their charms by our medicines. God has given us one little thing, which you know nothing of. He had given us the knowledge of certain medicines by which we can make rain, we do not despise those things which you possess, though we are ignorant of them, we don't understand your book, yet we don't despise it. You ought not to despise our little knowledge, though you are ignorant of it.

M.D.:	I don't despise what I am ignorant of; I only think you are mistaken in saying that you have medicines, which can influence the rain at all.
R.D.:	That's just the way people speak when they talk on a subject of which they have no knowledge. When we first opened our eyes, we found our forefathers making rain, and we follow in their footsteps. You, who send to Kuruman for corn, and irrigate your garden, may do without rain; we cannot manage in that way. If we had no rain, the cattle would have no pasture, the cows give no milk, our children become lean and die, our wives run away to other tribes who did make rain and have corn and the whole tribe become dispersed and lost; our fire would go out.
M.D.:	I quite agree with you as to the value of the rain; but you cannot charm the clouds by medicines. You wait till you see the clouds come, then you use your medicines, and take the credit which belongs to God only.
R.D.:	I use my medicines, and you employ yours; we are both doctors and doctors are not deceivers. You give a patient medicine. Sometimes God is pleased to heal him by means of your medicine; sometimes not—he dies. When he is cured, you take the credit of what God does. I do the same. Sometimes God grants us rain. When a patient dies, you don't give up trust in your medicine, neither do I when rain fails. If you wish

146

	me to leave off my medicine, why continue your own?
M.D.:	I give medicine to living creatures within my reach, and can see the effects, though no cure follows; you pretend to charm the clouds, which are so far above us that your medicines never reach them. The clouds usually lie in one direction, and your smoke goes in another. God alone can command the clouds. Only try and wait patiently; God alone will give us rain without your medicines.
R.D.:	Mahala-ma-kapa-a-a!! Well, I always thought white men were wise till this morning. Who ever thought of making a trial of starvation? Is death pleasant, then?
M.D.:	Could you make it rain on one spot and not on another?
R.D.:	I wouldn't think of trying, I like to see the whole country green, all the people glad; the women clapping their hands, and giving me their ornaments for thankfulness, and lullilooing for joy.
M.D.:	I think you deceive both them and yourself.
R.D.:	Well, then, there is a pair of us?[5]

Elling has also argued that although traditional medicine tends to be built upon accumulated understandings rather than on scientific proof, the bulk of Western medicine also shares this quality.[6] In conclusion, it is important to note that medical knowledge is part of culture. In other words, it is created within a cultural context and make sense in that context. The standards for evaluating the efficacy, the rationality, and the objectivity of a

147

particular form of medical knowledge is given by the medical communities within that culture. An examination of the exchange between the rain doctor and Livingstone shows that Livingstone claims superiority for his own form of medical knowledge based on the principle of empiricism.

Logical empiricism itself has been called into question by most contemporary philosophers of science. They reject the reduction of theoretical knowledge to empirical knowledge. Most important, they believe that knowledge does not begin with observations and sensual experience because observation is always preceded or attended by theoretical concepts.[7] It is precisely because Livingstone would not understand the theoretical apparatus and concepts of the rain doctor that forced him to erroneously place the rain doctor's practice within the context of his own theoretical apparatus.

Even the standard view of science and knowledge on which Livingstone based his condemnation of the rain doctor's practice has been successfully challenged by contemporary philosophers of science. Michael Mulkay, for example, had the following to say on the subject:

> The central assumption is that we can distinguish unambiguously between observing an object directly and merely inferring its characteristics from its effects. But seeing an object directly is thought to involve photons moving from the object in question as we think in these terms, the notion of direct observation starts to lose its clarity and thereby its usefulness, in separating fact from theory.[8]

And quoting Grandy, Mulkay continued saying that "if observability is merely a matter of degree, then there seems to be no plausible way of drawing a sharp line on this basis between objects which do and objects which do not exist."[9]

Efficacy

The claim of superiority of Western medicine over traditional medicine has also been made on the ground that the former is more efficacious for most health problems than traditional medicine. In this connection, a relevant question has been left unanswered or at best glossed over. Whose or what criterion should be used for judging efficacy? This question is important because there is no criterion given in nature for judging efficacy. Standards of efficacy are provided within theoretical systems which give an indication of what should be recognized as a problem, ways of solving problems so recognized, and what is to pass for solution.

It would seem therefore that efficacy ought to be seen not from the point of view of Western trained doctors who impose their acquired Western absolutist realities on those of utilizers of health services but from the point of view of the utilizers themselves. The utilizer's point of view gives as much credit to traditional as to Western medicine in terms of efficacy. One is of course aware that there are, aside from this, the purely technical problem of identification of active components, toxicity measurement, and dosage standardization in herbal remedies.

Elling's discussion of the issue presents a very balanced picture. Many specific measures and some programs of Western medicine are effective. For example, using antibiotic drugs to cure infections and eradicating diseases such as smallpox through inoculations. But it would be incorrect to attribute (as many people do) increased life expectancy since the last century in Europe to modern medicine. It also would be incorrect not to attribute beneficial impact from it. It is true that there is increasing demand for modern medicine, but at the same time there is increasing ambivalence regarding its complexity, impersonality, and its cost, and increasing uncertainty regarding its efficacy.

The situation in traditional medicine is similar. There are serious grounds for doubting the efficacy of much of it. At the same time, there are many proven examples of efficacious medicines and generally healthy practices embedded in it. The element of trust and confidence and humane support (the so-called placebo effect) may be more powerful in traditional than in Western medicine. The problem therefore is how to pick out the wheat from the chaff in both systems of medicine and from the result develop a humane system that can be sustained at successive levels of development. The attempts for underdeveloped countries in this regard should be, as China puts it, to "walk on two legs."

Cultural Hegemony and Underdevelopment of Traditional Medicine in Africa

In this section, I want to argue that the amount of support which traditional medicine receives at any point in time is a function of the existing power structures. In other words, there is a close relationship between the nature of the relationship between traditional and Western medicine and the political and economic structures of countries and their resource levels.

An important characteristic of underdeveloped countries is the coexistence of modern and traditional professions, both claiming to perform the same functions for society. But both do not receive the same kind of support from the ruling group in the society. The ruling group, the academic and political authorities, tend to accept the values of the modern professions and give their support to them with concomitant neglect or even outright suppression of the traditional professions. Consequently, the modern professions have higher status and state support and are therefore better developed while the repression and suppression of the traditional professions result in their underdevelopment. Janzen has documented the process of the underdevelopment of traditional medicine in Africa in this way. This process of underdevelopment started with contact with the West and indications are that it is continuing even under independent African governments. State power is the major vehicle for bringing together various strings and strands to form culture, including medical culture. But the state has become, as is often the case in capitalist oriented societies, an instrument in the hands of the ruling class. State power has been used particularly during colonial times and to a lesser degree since independence to viciously repress native cultures and the cultures of minorities.

The politics of culture is generally subtle but sometimes unashamedly repressive. At the level of the individual, Sherif's classic experiment shows how the exercise of power proceeds by removing ambiguities through the definition of the situation. Opinion leadership of the ruling elite in Africa is used in this manner. At the level of the state, Krause, following Gramsci's notion of cultural hegemony established by the ruling class, has demonstrated how cultural hegemony of the ruling class is established in medicine in the United States of America.[10]

Janzen has described the process by which cultural hegemony in medicine was imposed in Zaire. The situation he described is similar for most of colonized Africa:

> But colonial authorities had their own very strong notion of what African custom was and were repeatedly attempting to expurgate aberrations from it in the interest of keeping the colonized people's culture cohesive and orderly. The effect on concrete consultations was that diagnosis and divination with a prophet-seer was seen as conflict-arousing, prone to politicize the population, thus dangerous. Open consideration of witchcraft was punishable. Innocuous herbal treatment and bone setting was tolerated.[11]

Gish said of Africa, Asia, and the America, colonized by Europe:

> The conquest of Asia, Africa and the Americas by Europe and the consequent assumption of state power by Europeans led to the virtual world-wide domination of European forms of organisation and scientific systems. Western medicine, like virtually all other things European, received official support while traditional systems either received none or were consciously suppressed.[12]

The governments of most of the ex-colonies on achieving independence have continued largely in this manner. The elites in these countries adopted virtually unchanged the instruments as well as the attitudes, perceptions, and values of the colonial governments. Thus in Nigeria, for example, independent governments, among other things, went on to multiply the number of Government Reserved Areas (GRAs) in the country and continued even more stridently than the colonial officers in the denigration of the traditional systems of medicine.

There is sufficient evidence that the ruling elite in underdeveloped capitalist countries ensures for itself access to Western medicine. It is argued that this preference for Western medicine cannot be explained by the simple fact that it appears to be more efficacious for a greater number of illness than traditional medicine, particularly in view of the fact that the issue of efficacy, as we have noted, is full of ambiguities. Janzen suggests that a more pertinent explanation also will need to take into account the consonance between class and care.

> Modern medicine is technologically and scientifically based as is the industrial society itself. Its knowledge is disguised as esoteric whereas folk medicine is widely shared. It tends to be elitist and hierarchical with physicians at the top . . . it can be more easily controlled by the ruling class than can a popularly based form of health care.
>
> Traditional medicine by contrast . . . is more generally the province of everyone with less concentration in the hands of experts; it is more dependent upon or works through social support in the community; and it is relatively inexpensive.[13]

Consequently, in nonsocialist societies, the traditional medicine which is available may be of poor quality because of its general subordinate position and exclusion from an organized system.

Elling has postulated that the mix of traditional and Western medicine that prevails in any country is determined by the political and economic structures and the resources level (Table 1). Obviously, most African countries fell into the group of capitalist-oriented countries with low resource base. Their medical systems therefore provide Western medicine for the elite and under-developed traditional medicine and some extremely poor quality Western medicine for the peasants and workers. Is the situation as it is today acceptable? For a number of reasons it is not. In the first place, a situation which does not provide the opportunity for the development and actualization of the potentials in traditional medicine, and instead actively destroys it, does a great disservice to mankind. In the second place, it is not acceptable because, as Brownrigg has warned, every whole culture lost through repression, represents a loss in the human's species past, and a loss of alternatives for organization of future societies.[14] The ethnobotany of the people also gets lost in the process. Depletion of culture is thus like the depletion of natural resources, once gone, always gone.

The present situation is also not acceptable from a purely pragmatic, practical, and utilitarian position. A good number of items in the traditional pharmacopoeia and a large number of the medical techniques are efficacious. These represent sources of medical treatment that should not be further underdeveloped, but rather developed and utilized more systematically and widely. This is particularly so given the low resource base from which most African countries are developing. Is it possible to create a situation in African countries which will make it possible to begin the process of actualizing the potentials in traditional medicine? The answer of course is yes.

Table 1

MIXES OF TRADITIONAL AND WESTERN MEDICINE

Political-Economic System	Resources	
	Low	High
Socialist-oriented	Merger of traditional and Western medicine, with system made generally available (China).	Western medicine predominates with system made generally available (Cuba, USSR).
Capitalist-oriented	Western medicine the ruling class, traditional medicine of poor quality for the peasants and working class (India, Mexico, Zaire, Nigeria, Ghana).	Western medicine predominates but unequally distributed in favor of ruling class. What traditional medicine there is, is more employed by the working class (US, UK). Both Western and traditional medicine for working class of poor quality.

In the remaining part of this chapter, I will examine the issues involved in the coexistence of medical systems and sub-systems and suggest a pattern of coexistence which I believe will be beneficial for all of Africa. Cross-cultural comparison of medical systems abound in the literature. Only a few of the studies available are geared specifically toward the practical problem of how to ensure that the populations of the Third World countries which have plural medical systems are enabled to get maximum benefits from the available systems. Recently more literature geared toward this goal has been emerging.

Aside from this practical utilization consideration, there is the possibility that there could be yet undiscovered invaluable knowledge in the traditional medicines of Africa merely waiting to be discovered and made widely and systematically available. Most governments of developing countries have attitudes toward traditional medicine which are not helpful in the effort to ensure their better utilization, and which therefore hinder the efforts to research into them and promote unawareness that this is beginning to change in countries like Nigeria, Ghana, Zambia, and Ethiopia. There is beginning to appear an improved attitude toward traditional medicine. In 1985, for example, the government of Lagos State in Nigeria allowed traditional healers to take part in health care delivery in an officially recognized setting. The modalities are still being worked out. The federal government of Nigeria in the same year set up a panel to work out how to utilize "alternative medicine" in official health care delivery. On 27 January 1985, it was announced that The International Confederation of Natural Alternative Medicine Associations (CIANAN) is to train practitioners of alternative medicine.[15] The World Health Organization (WHO) also reported that with UNDP support it collaborated with Ethiopia in 1982-1983 to bring traditional medicine into its national health system and started a training program for traditional practitioners.[16] In the same period, Zambia created a traditional medicine unit in its ministry of health, while professional associations of traditional healers were organized in Benin, Cameroon, Congo, and Ghana, among others.

By 1983, WHO had sixteen centers all over the world (of which four were in Africa) which collaborate to strengthen national efforts in research on and development of traditional medicine. Results of activities from various parts of the continent indicate that the hopes may not be misplaced. For example, at Obafemi Awolowo University in Nigeria, the Unit for Plant Research and the Development of African Pharmacopoeia among other achievements has discovered *Fagora zenthoxyloides* in *Orin-ata*, a Yoruba chewing stick, to be effective in the treatment of sickle-cell anemia. The department has also tested the substance for toxicity and provided dosage specifications. The University of Benin Pharmacy Department (also in Nigeria) is now to produce the drug in tablet form.[17] Similarly, the West African Pharmaceutical Federation (WSPF) reported that doctors working at the Scientific Research Centre into Plant Medicine, located at Mampong Ghana, have processed cryptoleine, an alkaloid with strong antimicrobial activity from a traditional Ghanian herbal treatment for malaria and rheumatism.[18]

The remaining part of this essay will focus on the coexistence of medical systems; clarify the issues involved, and recommend a pattern that is likely to ensure better use and development of traditional medicine. Traditional medicine may be defined as the system of health care (preventive, curative, health maintenance), as understood and practiced by indigenous peoples uninfluenced by Western medicine.[19] Before contact with the West, the various socio-cultural groups in Africa developed their own systems of medicine. These comprised a world view and ideas as to the case of illness from which preventive, curative, and health maintenance techniques were derived. The Yoruba, for example, have a system based on the role of the *Babalawo* and *Onisegun*, the Hausa one based on the role of the herbalist, among others. The barber-surgeon, the Koranic Mallam, and the Urhobo had a system based on the role of the *Obo*.

In Africa and most underdeveloped nations it is unfashionable in medical circles to talk positively about traditional medicine. The assumption seems to be that there is very little worth in the traditional system. The majority of Western-type health personnel therefore close-mindedly dismiss traditional systems as a load of old rubbish. Yet those of them who have taken time to look more deeply but critically have found that there is indeed something of worth in spite of their many undesirable aspects. A context needs to be created to bring out, enhance, and systematically utilize this worth.

Possible Patterns of Coexistence

The major dimensions of medical systems are drugs and medicines, healing techniques, manpower, and medical concepts and paradigms. Coexistence of systems becomes increasingly difficult as one moves from drugs and medicine through healing techniques to concepts and paradigms.

Structured or unstructured coexistence of medical systems and subsystems could exist. The coexistence would be structured if it was deliberately regulated in some way by rules and regulations; it would be unstructured if there were no rules and regulations. Structured coexistence could take the form of structured competition, structured cooperation, and integration.

Structured Competition. This has been defined as two or more medical systems legally regulated and supervised which compete for the same secondary medical resources in society.[20] Primary medical resources are drugs, healing techniques, equipment, and facilities, and may be differentiated from secondary medical resources which are material and non-material rewards that accrue to practitioners of medicine through their practice.

Structured competition may be better than nonstructured competition, yet it is undesirable because the primary medical resources of the systems in competition with each other may not be equally suited to tackle effectively the total range of health problems of the people. Moreover, because they are in competition, practitioners in either system find that it is not to their advantage to admit the limitations and weakness of their primary resources for certain applications. One of the implications of such competition is that patients may ignorantly resort to one system only to find its primary resources unable to cope. The patient may then resort to the competing systems. The consequence of this is loss of valuable time which creates room for the problem to get more complicated.

The medical situation in most of Africa today reflects such competition. Traditional practitioners are allowed to practice but under severely crippling and limiting laws. Coupled with this is an ongoing campaign, sometimes overt, mostly subtle, to discredit traditional practitioners and discourage the people from utilizing their services. Western medical practitioners and most government policymakers see the traditional systems as nothing but quackery and mumbo-jumbo while traditional practitioners see Western medical practitioners as enemies and look on government functionaries with suspicion. As we said earlier, happily this situation is beginning to change.

Structured cooperation. In this form of coexistence a formal referral system in both directions exists. Competition for patients patronage is made unnecessary and the mode and contents of training of practitioners ensures that each is able and willing to recognize the possibilities and limitations of his own and other systems and to act accordingly.[21] This kind of cooperation is possible in all four dimensions of medical systems—drugs, healing techniques, manpower, and concepts and paradigms.

I want to argue, following Unschuld, that it is difficult to practice structured cooperation in situations where health is regarded as a free-market commodity. In such a situation, certain interests such as those of multinational drug companies and the practitioners of Western medicine may be dependent on the predominance of the Western system rather than on the traditional. These interests will ensure that such attempts at cooperation fail. The situation is even more difficult for Third World countries such as Nigeria, given their underdeveloped nature and structure. China is the only country where this kind of cooperation has been achieved. Such achievement is not surprising as such cooperation operates better in a socialist framework; it requires an open mind on the part of policymakers and a willingness to experiment.

Integration. Integration is the progressive end of the scale of structured coexistence. Where it has been achieved, we cease to speak of different or distinct medical systems of subsystems. Integration is achievable and has been achieved with respect to drugs and healing techniques. Drugs such as quinine, ephedrine, and techniques such as acupuncture are cases in point. With respect to manpower, confusion often exists between subordination and integration. When most people talk of integration, they in fact mean the subordination of traditional medical practitioners to practitioners of Western medicine. Traditional medical practitioners are to be paramedical personnel or auxiliaries to Western practitioners. This should not surprise anyone. As we had said earlier, the policymakers and professionals were trained in the Western mode and they have interests of a material and non-material nature to protect. The influence of Western medical men who successfully propagated the caricature of traditional medicine painted by Una Maclean constitutes a valuable economic and political resource for the capitalist Western world and officials in national government who from narrow selfish interest act by and large as agents or collaborators.[22]

What we refer to as integration here is the situation where all relevant primary medical resources are equally accessible to the previously different manpower groups with specialization occurring on the same basis as it occurs in Western medicine. China at one time attempted to implement such integration but abandoned it for a policy of structured cooperation. Vietnam also attempted to implement a policy of integration.

Recommended Pattern of Coexistence

In the literature, suggestions as to how traditional and Western medicine should coexist are varied. For example, Oke suggested the integration of successful traditional drugs into Western medical practice in Nigeria.[23] This sort of integration has been done in other places as the examples given earlier show and is similar to the suggestion by the Nigerian National Council on Health. In our view, selective acceptance is unprogressive as it involves merely borrowing a few medicaments from traditional medicine to enrich the primary resources of Western medicine while neglecting the practice of traditional medicine. This is not to say that the medicaments used in traditional medical treatment do not require study and refinement and standardization.

Harrison focused on personnel and suggested the integration of traditional healers into Western medical practice after a period of retraining.[24] Again, such a practice would be unprogressive as it implies allowing traditional systems of medicine to decline as their personnel are gradually absorbed into Western medical practice.

While these two suggestions are unlikely to be wholly unfruitful, it is our view that it will be more beneficial for the populations of Africa who need all the varied services and for the general state of knowledge of mankind if African countries attempt to achieve structured cooperation as the pattern of coexistence between traditional and Western medicine. Endorsement by WHO has encouraged an examination of the value of traditional medicine in most developing countries from which new cultural awareness and pride in traditional values have emerged.[25] The important thing is not to allow this new found national pride to fizzle out but translate it into meaningful form of action. In this respect, WHO has also given the lead which I believe will produce useful results if followed by African governments. The WHO program is composed of three lines of action which are meant to proceed simultaneously. These are (a) evaluation of traditional materia medica and practices, (b) making traditional medicine a part of the national health care system, and (c) training.[26]

Evaluation of traditional practices is meant to help separate myth from reality in traditional medicine and to ensure that valid practices and remedies can be separated from those that are ineffective and or unsafe. WHO is continuously developing analytic methods for doing this in its various collaborating countries, five of which are in Africa. It would be in the interest of all African people if governments, universities, and relevant national organizations in Africa were to cooperate in the work of these collaborating centers.

Traditional Medicine as Part of the National Health Care System

While evaluation efforts are continuing, national governments in Africa should start to make traditional medicine part of the national health care system rather than paying lip service to the idea. Structured cooperation as I have suggested would require training on two fronts.

Conventional health workers should be shown the traditional health practices and remedies which have proven safe and effective. Traditional practitioners on the other hand, should be given additional skills so that they can become allies rather than competitors with practitioners of allopathic medicine. For example, they would be trained in such beneficial practices as simple hygiene and asepsis and modern methods of prevention and care of infants with diarrhoea. Traditional birth attendants could be trained in aseptic delivery techniques and sample antenatal and postpartum care. Herbalists could be trained in the standardization of plant extracts used in treatment.

Apart from these lines of action one may mention specifically the need to use plants as alternative sources of scarce drugs for primary health care. Plants have been a common source of medicaments either in the form of traditional preparations or extracts of

159

their active principles. Decision makers in Africa therefore need to identify locally available plants or plant extracts which could be added to the list of useful drugs and which perhaps could replace some imported pharmaceutical preparations.

This pattern of coexistence would be beneficial for a number of reasons. It would make available to the population in a more organized way the varieties of treatments available in both the traditional and Western medicine. It would ensure that knowledge available in both systems are preserved and improved for the benefit of all mankind. It would enable each system to specialize in the treatment of the problem it is best equipped to treat and avoid the waste of unnecessary competition between the two systems. Finally, it would enhance the expansion of badly needed health delivery facilities.

NOTES

1. D. N. Ojanuga, "What Doctors Think of Traditional Healers and Vice-Versa," *World Health Forum* 2 (1981): 47.
2. For a comprehensive review, see S. K. Bonsi, "Traditional Medical Practices in Modern Ghana," Ph.D. Diss., University of Missouri, 1973, chapter 1.
3. R. Horton, "African Traditional Thought and Western Science" in *Rationality*, ed. B. R. Wilson (Worcester: Basil Blackwell, 1984), chapter 4.
4. J. M. Janzen, *The Quest for Therapy in Lower Zaire* (Berkeley: University of California Press, 1978). See also J. Powels, "On the Limitations of Modern Medicine," *Science, Medicine and Man* 1 (1973).
5. Janzen, *Quest*, pp. 97-98.
6. R. H. Elling, "Political Economy, Cultural Hegemony, and Mixes of Traditional and Modern Medicine," *Social Science and Medicine* 158 (1981): 89-99.
7. I. Naletov, *Alternatives to Positivism* (Moscow: Progress Publishers, 1984), pp. 9-11.
8. M. Mulkay, *Science and the Sociology of Knowledge* (London: George Allen and Unwin, 1979), pp. 30-31. See also P. Berger and T. Luckman, *The Social Construction of Reality: A Treatise on the Sociology of Knowledge* (New York: Doubleday, 1967).
9. Mulkay, *Science*, p. 31; cited from R. B. Grandy, *Theories and Observation in Science* (Englewood Cliffs, Prentice Hall, 1973), p. 71.
10. E. A. Krause, *Power and Illness: The Political Sociology of Health and Medical Care* (New York: Elsevier, 1977).
11. Janzen, *Quest*, pp. 14-15.
12. Cited in Elling, "Political Economy." See U. Gish, "The Political Economy of Primary Care and 'Health by the

161

People': An Historical Explanation," *Social Science and Medicine* 13c (1979): 203-11.

13. Janzen, *Quest*, p. 96.
14. L. A. Brownrigg, "Repression Stops the Progress of Native Culture in Paraguay," *WIN* 12 (1976).
15. *Sunday New Nigerian*, January 27, 1985. On the attitude of the Nigerian government to traditional medicine, see the address given by the Commissioner for Health, Lagos State, Mrs. K. Pratt to the International Symposium on Traditional Medical Therapy, in *Proceedings of the International Symposium on Traditional Medical Therapy* (Lagos: University of Lagos, 1973), the address given by the Military Governor of Lagos State in the same publication, and the minutes of the interview between the Commissioner for Health and the representatives of the Central Executive Committee of the Midwest Central Union of Herbalists, June 1972, Ministry of Health File HA 149, Vol. IV.
16. *WHO Chronicle* 38 (1984): 76-81.
17. *The Guardian*, 29 January 1985.
18. *Sunday Times*, 3 March 1985.
19. Paul Unschuld, "Western Medicine and Traditional Healing Systems: Cooperation or Integration," *Ethics, Science and Medicine* 3 (May 1976).
20. Unschuld, "Western Medicine," p. 9.
21. Unschuld, "Western Medicine," p. 9.
22. Una Maclean, *Magical Medicine: A Nigerian Case Study* (London: Penguin, 1971).
23. O. I. Oke, "Probable Theory of the Efficacy of Traditional Medicine," *Proceedings of the International Symposium on Traditional Medical Therapy* (Lagos: University of Lagos, 1973): 18-42.
24. I. H. Harrison, "Traditional Healers: A Neglected Source of Health Manpower," *Proceedings of the International Symposium on Traditional Medical Therapy*, pp. 14-22.
25. O. Akerele, "WHO's Traditional Medicine Programme: Progress and Perspective," *WHO Chronicle* 38/2 (1984): 76-81.
26. Akerele, "WHO's Traditional Medicine Program," pp. 76-81.

9

VIOLENCE, CONFLICT, AND HEALTH IN AFRICA

Dennis A. Ityavyar and Leo O. Ogba

Violence and conflict have become almost daily experiences in Africa. These upheavals include civil wars, peasant uprisings, religious riots, student demonstrations, and labor unrest. Between 1960 and 1987 no less than sixteen African countries were involved in violence and political conflicts. Examples of these include Zaire, Mauritania, Algeria, Morocco, Ethiopia, Somalia, Kenya, Sudan, Chad, and Nigeria in the 1960s and Zimbabwe, Uganda, Tanzania, Angola, and Mozambique in the 1970s and 1980s. Several countries in Africa such as Chad, Angola, and Ethiopia have engaged in civil wars. Other recurring cases of violence occurred because of religious disturbances such as those in Nigeria and Sudan, violent student demonstrations in Liberia, Ghana, and Buckin a Fasso, labor and civil unrest in South Africa. In this chapter, we examine the consequences of violence and conflicts on the development of health services and health policy in Africa.

Violence, Conflicts, and Health

Violence and conflicts have specific impacts on health care policies through increases in military spending that negate health care priorities through physical destruction of social infrastructures such as hospitals, roads, and industrial activities, all of which have substantial impact in the formulation of long-term health policies and because of refugee problems which create constant mobility of displaced persons by wars and other political violence, exacerbate problems of hunger and malnutrition and what sometimes create long-term health problems.

163

The biennial report of the director general to the World Health Organization Assembly and the United Nations in 1984 focused on violence and conflict as they affect African health care. The report unequivocally confirmed that many African states still living through periods of civil wars and the destabilization policies of the South African apartheid system have experienced material and human damage which perpetuate their poverty and indirectly affect health care policies.[1] The WHO report further emphasized that funds used by South Africa's neighboring countries to preserve their economic and political independence as well as to cater to the acute increase of refugee movements across their borders cannot be put at the service of indispensable health development efforts of these nations. These many aspects of insecurity caused by violence and conflicts in the African region certainly must affect WHO's pronouncement of health for all by the year 2000. To examine more critically the extent to which cases of violence and conflicts affect health care policies in Africa, we have chosen for analysis at least seventeen conflicts that occurred in the period 1960-1987. These examples will enable us to draw conclusions concerning how violence related to underdevelopment of health services in Africa.

Conflicts and wars have become constant fratricidal escapades for most African states since the raging fire of colonization caught up with most Africans. The post independence era has seen no improvement in the sad situation. However, our view of violence and conflict as used in this study covers only events in which African states engaged each other in confrontations in which there was use of force; conflicts or violence in which African Liberation Forces were seeking consistently to assert control or sovereignty over a particular territory in Africa and in which large scale or limited use of force was applied against the colonial authorities involved; and violent events in which rival groups or insurgent forces within one state abandoned the political processes to use organized and prolonged military means to change the structure of power within a particular state.[2]

The scale of forces, mobility of persons, and the disruption of infrastructure that normally accompany the category of violence and conflict considered here were considerable enough to affect public policy as will be considered later in the case of health. The taxonomy of violence and conflicts considered here is exhaustive and fairly represent the types of conflicts that have occurred in African states.

For the purpose of the present study, coup d'etats and minor diplomatic disruptions between states, unless they were accompanied by social upheaval carrying the possibility of escalation and wide conflict, have been considered in our view as not serious. Although coup d'etats are becoming a common feature of the African political scene, their direct impact on public policy of African states cannot be generalized easily.[3] Violence also includes activities that disturb peace such as religious riots and student demonstrations.

Independent African states have witnessed incessant conflicts with serious social consequences. Shortly after independence in 1960, the Congo (Zaire) erupted into a major civil war and set Africa on a major path of disequilibrium. Since that period Zaire has been forced into a series of other debilitating crises. Each time, the state abandoned pressing social development to concentrate on consolidation of sovereignty. In addition, the massive refugee situation generated by the Zairean conflicts affected other African states, especially neighboring Angola, Uganda, and Tanzania. The experience of Zaire has been duplicated in other African conflicts that have occurred in Ethiopia, Chad, Angola, Zaire, Sudan, Somalia, Burundi, Nigeria, Zimbabwe, and South Africa.

The conflicts in Ethiopia, Somalia, and Eritrea have been responsible for the building up of the largest military reserves in Africa at least in number of personnel. As a result of Ethiopia's wars with its neighbors, its military force rose from 2,500 in 1963 to 250,000 in 1982.[4] At the same time the conflict in the Horn of Africa has been responsible for the high influx of refugees in that region since 1963. The Ethiopia-Somalia war has affected more than 1.5 million refugees. The Eritrean conflict alone produced 350,000 refugees between 1979 and 1981, most of whom were forced to seek asylum in Sudan.[5]

Between 1965 and 1987 Chad was torn by incessant conflicts. The state became militarized and a thriving front for France, USA, and Libya, each country providing military aid with the view of exercising dominant influence. Chad remains one of the five poorest states of the world with very little investment in social policies. Extensive military assistance from France, Libya, and more recently, the United States continues to fuel the Chadian conflict.

Refugees have been a constant burden to Chad's neighbors, notably Nigeria, Cameroon, and Sudan. Between 1981 and 1982, the members of the Organization of African Unity (OAU) raised about $236.71 million to maintain the OAU peace force in Chad. It is interesting, incidentally, that this was more than the total fund which Chad allocated to health care in ten years. Nigeria's share of $62.9 million spent in the peace-keeping operation to Chad was almost the equivalent of the national health allocation for the 1981 fiscal year.[6]

Sudan and Burundi are the other African states which have experienced internal violence since 1961. Even though conflicts have erupted intermittently, refugee problems have been more constant. Many people from the Tutsi and Hutu ethnic groups of Burundi have been forced to flee into Rwanda and Uganda. In Sudan, Christians of the South continue a war of attrition and social deprivation with the government. While military spending and military policies have been given some priority in Sudan, the country continues to depend on international assistance to support domestic policies.[7]

The Nigerian Civil War between 1967 and 1970 remains one of the fiercest internal conflicts in Africa, both in its human toll and in social costs. During this war Nigeria's defence spending increased remarkably while social spending decreased. Social infrastructure including hospitals, roads, and industries were virtually destroyed, especially in the secessionist Biafra. In 1966 only 6.8 percent (₦29m) of the national budget was devoted to defence. This rose to 24.1 percent (₦162m) in 1968 when the civil war started. As the war continued, the defence budget rose to 32.3 percent (₦359m) in 1969 and 42.6 percent (₦314m) by 1970. In the same period health expenditure fell from 3.7 percent (₦6.2m) in 1967 to .8 percent (₦3.9m) in 1969 and 1.1 percent (₦6.1m) in 1970.[8] The mass destruction of hospitals and clinics was accompanied with the most glaring problem of the more than two million refugees created by the war.

Between 1976 and 1984, and before the Western Sahara declared itself an independent state of the Saharawi Arab Republic (SADR), Morocco was involved with the Western Sahara Liberation Movement (POLISARO) in a protracted war over Western Sahara. During this period, more than 70,000 refugees fled from the disputed territory into the neighboring states of Mauritania and

Senegal. Yet to carry on the war in the Western Sahara, Morocco's military spending between 1978 and 1984 averaged between 16 percent and 18 percent of gross government yearly expenditures; the same time the rising price of food was causing intermittent riots in different cities of Morocco.[9]

In Mozambique also, violent activities of South African supported rebels—Mozambique National Resistance (MNR)—caused untold damage to the policies of the socialist state in Mozambique. Rebel incursions not only resulted in an insecurity dilemma in Mozambique and increased military spending, but the rebels have prevented Mozambique farmers from cultivating crops and the national government from distributing seeds to millions of farmers.[10] The result of such rebel activities was that millions of Mozambiquans in 1987 were reported to be facing imminent death through starvation.[11]

The Academic Staff Union of Universities (ASUU) recounted a case of violence at Ahmadu Bello University at Zaria in Nigeria involving police and students where between twenty and thirty people were killed, many people injured, and much property destroyed.[12] A recent event in this category of violence was religious disturbances in Kaduna state of Nigeria in March 1987. The violence involved a clash between Moslems and Christians and resulted in many injuries and the loss of many lives. More than 100 churches were burnt down during the disturbance. Property such as houses and cars was also destroyed. Riots such as these have implications for health services in Africa.[13] All those disasters and social consequences noted here were not made by Nature but were political and could have been resolved through political decisions. They had direct consequences on the health policies of African states as we illustrate below.

Using African conflicts and violence as conceived here, we have tried to address the following questions:

1.   Do African conflicts and violence increase the military spending of the affected states? Is so, how do these relate to health care policies?

2.   How can damage resulting from wars and violence in Africa affect long-term health care programming in African states?

3.   Can the reduction in the numbers of war refugees in Africa improve health care services of host and affected states?

167

4. Is a regional policy of conflict reduction in Africa of any relevance to health care policies?

Violent activities lead to serious implications for health services development in Africa. First, it leads to uncontrolled defence expenditures to the neglect of the social sector. Second, as earlier stated, victims of violence are often treated in hospitals by medical professionals with drugs and equipment which could have been put to a better use.

As a result of violence and conflicts in which refugee problems have become a feature of the African continent, new pressure on the social policies of states has emerged. The council of ministers of the Organization of African Unity recognized this problem when it noted:

> One thing that is clear is that the concept of African traditional hospitality which has enabled hundreds of thousands of African refugees to find asylum in many African countries, has reached a saturation point. Unless the refugee exporting countries look more seriously at the human toll, the misery and the loss and wastage of human and material resources involved, we run the calculated risk of getting used to an *ugly* situation in Africa.[14]

Human waste, superfluous military spending, and the problem of refugees are issues related to violence and conflict in the past three decades in Africa (Table 1).

Military Spending and Health Policies of African States

Defense expenditure has increased spectacularly over the years as African armies emerged from the rubble of security forces in the colonial period. African armies have become more expensive and more destructive, and their expenditures have become three times as great in real terms of what they were in the 1960s.[15] These massive increases in expenditures and in the size of African armies can be related to four main factors. These are an increase in national resources and perceived security needs, the threat of violence, and involvement in conflict. In most instances,

Table 1

MILITARY EXPENDITURES OF AFRICAN STATES 1963 AND 1977-1980: A COMPARISON (in millions $US)*

Country	1963	1977	1978	1979	1980
Algeria	66.0	471	527	602	705
Benin (Dahomey)	1.1	9	10	16	22
Botswana	-	-	15	27	33
Burundi	1.2	13	21	25	35
Cameroon	15.0	50	55	88	82
Central African Republic	2.1	9	10	14	13
Chad	1.5	24	37	40	22
Congo Brazzaville	3.7	36	34	52	61
Equatorial Guinea	-	5	6	6	6
Ethiopia	17.9	135	159	349	447
Gabon	2.5	18	49	69	74
Ghana	35.3	42	60	60	50
Guinea	5.8	21	23	-	9
Ivory Coast	8.7	60	79	98	125
Kenya	6.0	148	189	291	100
Liberia	2.1	7	9	13	26
Libya	14.0	140	439	500	503
Madagascar	9.0	43	47	82	94
Malawi	-	15	23	47	55
Mauritania	4.0	11	28	38	39
Morocco	93.0	731	326	396	1,120
Mozambique	-	49	83	114	160
Niger	34.0	8	8	12	17
Nigeria	28.0	1,964	2,040	1,991	2,288
Senegal	9.0	44	56	59	64
Sierra Leone	2.2	6	7	8	14
Somalia	3.9	12	40	95	105
South Africa	219.0	2,138	2,185	2,269	2,320
Sudan	21.5	228	216	199	200
Tanzania	1.3	133	172	267	250
Togo	4.0	16	19	23	23

*The dollar value used in this table is not constant. Values expressed for each year represent dollar prices at the ruling exchange rate for the years.

Country	1963	1977	1978	1979	1980
Tunisia	11.4	160	185	363	337
Uganda	1.5	97	146	161	125
Upper Volta(Burkina Faso)	2.8	22	27	32	35
Zaire	10	155	263	110	200
Zambia	-	360	223	294	516
Zimbabwe	-	293	221	427	478

Sources: Compiled from Ruth L. Sivard, *World Military and Social Expenditures, 1980-1983* (Washington: World Priorities); and George Weeks, "The Armies of Africa," *Africa Report* 9 (January 1963): 3-21. See also, L. O. Ogba, *Emerging Patterns of Conflict Management*, p. 317.

the growing size of African armies and their military spending have failed to buy security. The implication is that most African countries that have experienced great change in military spending and army strength are either preparing to play an active part in existing conflicts in their region or are recovering from recent involvement.

Between 1963 and 1982, African states that were involved with violence and conflict showed dramatic changes in their military strength. Among such countries were Algeria, Ethiopia, Libya, Morocco, Nigeria, Somalia, Sudan, Tanzania, Zaire, Zimbabwe, and South Africa (Table 1). All such increases in military strength were accompanied by the massive importation of arms and concomitant waste of national resources. For example, between 1977 and 1979, as a result of the Ethiopian-Somalia conflict, both states spent more on arms imports (more than 10 percent of their national income) than did all the Nordic countries plus the Netherlands.[16]

The strength of most African armies as well as military expenditures and military consumption of national resources increased dramatically in the period between 1963 and 1982 (Tables 1 and 2). This period also coincides with the era of escalating conflicts in Africa. However, the link between military consumption of resources and health care priorities is less clear. One reason for this must be related to the fact that most analysts cannot agree that funds from reduced military spending can be transferred to improved social spending, especially health.

170

Table 2
CHANGES IN AFRICAN MILITARY POWER:
A COMPARISON, 1963-1982*

Country	Military Forces 1963		1982		Average Military Exp. as % of Central Govt. Exp. 1975-1982	
Algeria	48,000	(1)	101,000	(4)	7.6	(19)
Benin	1,000	(19)	3,150	(30)	15.3	(10)
Burundi	800	(30)	5,200	(25)	22.2	(10)
Burkina Faso	1,000	(19)	3,700	(28)	18.2	(7)
Cameroon	2,700	(12)	7,300	(20)	19.9	(16)
Cent. African Rep.	500	(22)	2,300	(31)	8.9	(18)
Chad	400	(23)	4,200	(27)	n/a	
Congo Brazzaville	700	(21)	8,700	(18)	14.4	(11)
Ethiopia	2,500	(13)	250,000	(1)	42.6	(1)
Gabon	700	(21)	3,200	(29)	1.1	(26)
Gambia	none		475		0.0	
Ghana	8,000	(5)	12,600	(15)	3.7	(24)
Guinea	4,800	(7)	9.900	(16)	n/a	
Ivory Coast	4,000	(9)	5,070	(21)	3.6	(25)
Kenya	2,500	(15)	16,000	(13)	12.9	(13)
Liberia	3,500	(10)	5,520	(24)	5.1	(21)
Libya	5,000	(6)	53,000	(7)	4.5	(23)
Malagasy Republic	2,600	(14)	21,100	(12)	13.5	(12)
Mali	3,100	(11)	4,650	(26)	20.5	(5)
Mauritania	500	(22)	8,170	(19)	25.9	(2)
Morocco	34,000	(2)	117,000	(3)	17.8	(8)
Niger	1,200	(18)	2,150	(32)	4.8	(22)
Nigeria	8,000	(5)	133,000	(2)	9.3	(17)
Senegal	1,850	(17)	9,700	(17)	11.4	(15)
Somalia	4,600	(8)	62,550	(6)	18.4	(6)
Sudan	11,000	(4)	68,000	(5)	12.2	(14)
Tanzania	2,000	(15)	40,000	(9)	16.3	(9)
Togo	250	(24)	5,080	(23)	7.0	(20)
Tunisia	20,000	(3)	29,000	(10)	4.5	(23)
Uganda	2,000	(16)	15,000	(14)	20.6	(4)

*The ranking for each state in this comparison is given in parentheses.

Country	Military Forces 1963		Military Forces 1982		Average Military Exp. as % of Central Govt. Exp. 1975-1982	
Zaire	n/a		42,000	(8)	12.4	(14)
Zimbabwe	0		24,000	(11)	29.9	(2)
South Africa	25,000	(3)	78,000	(5)	13.9	(12)

Sources: *The Military Balance* (1970-1984) (London: International Institute of Strategic Studies); George Weeks, "The Armies of Africa," *Africa Report*, January 1964, pp. 4-21.

Table 3

INCREASE ON MILITARY AND HEALTH EXPENDITURE
1972-1978 BY COUNTRY

	States	Defense (%)	Health (%)
1.	Chad	28.2	3.9
2.	Botswana	10.3	6.0
3.	Burkina Faso	30.4	3.3
4.	Burundi	12.0	3.6
5.	Ethiopia	42.6	4.2
6.	Ghana	4.7	7.5
7.	Ivory Coast	7.5	7.7
8.	Kenya	20.5	7.2
9.	Liberia	1.6	4.6
10.	Malawi	15.1	5.1
11.	Mauritius	0.4	7.6
12.	Nigeria	14.6	2.0
13.	Sierra Leone	14.9	11.4
14.	Somalia	17.9	5.3
15.	Sudan	9.5	0.2
16.	Tanzania	10.2	5.7
17.	Zambia	-	8.3

Source: Compiled from The World Bank, *Accelerated Development in Sub-Sahara Africa, An Agenda for Action* (Washington: World Bank, 1983), p. 185.

Countries (such as Ethiopia) which are involved in conflict, or are recovering from conflict, characteristically have high defense spending and low social expenditures, especially in the health sector during the same period (Table 3).

Between 1972 and 1978 when the Chadian conflict was raging increases on defense rose by 28.2 percent, while health rose only by 3.9. Also in Somalia during the same period, defense increases rose by 17.9 percent.[17] Other African states such as Burundi, Tanzania, and Nigeria which were either directly involved in conflict or played an active role in regional conflict equally showed a high priority given to defense with less regard for health funding. Almost all the African countries that were not involved in some form of violence or conflict experienced a more balanced growth in defense and health expenditure. These occurred without regard to the nature of the regime in power—whether military or civilian. For example, the Ivory Coast, Mauritius, Liberia, and Ghana all experienced a low but uniform growth in defense spending and a slightly higher growth in health allocations during the years between 1972 and 1978. These states were also relatively free from internal violence and external conflicts. The relatively stable states of Kenya and Sierra Leone both experienced a rise in defense spending between 1972 and 1978 which corresponded with the same high emphasis on improved health care allocation.

It is important to note here that increases in defense expenditures even in countries free from internal violence and external conflicts shows an emerging trend of the position of the military in African politics. In many African countries top military officers are part of the ruling class and control the government. As a result they have considerable influence on state policy especially in the defense sector where they derive direct benefits, for example in comparatively high salaries.

The importance of the military in politics also has led to an increase in the size of the officer corps. Beside her large number of officers, Nigeria now has many retired military generals who still draw salaries from the Ministry of Defense. This, added to the rapid promotion in the army, leads to increased budgetary allocation to the defense sector. Expenditures in the defense sector are not only for weapons; sometimes a larger expenditure is for salaries and allowances. For these reasons countries, such as Ivory Coast, who have not experienced any violence or conflicts, still have increasing defense expenditures. We now turn to a discussion of how violence influences health policies in Africa.

Violence and Health Policy

Conflicts and violence have direct effects on the health policies of African states. Existing health infrastructure destroyed in riots and conflicts often have to be replaced. Attention of policymakers is diverted from other areas of health care that otherwise would be the focus of health policy. The physical destruction of hospitals, dispensaries, clinics, and personnel such as doctors affect health policy as it does not give room for growth and development in the health sector. In African countries (such as Chad and Angola) involved in war, new health policies first must take cognisance of infrastructure destroyed by war before replacement may be considered.

The use of medical services to treat soldiers and other victims of political conflicts convinces policymakers in such countries to consolidate their policies based upon the medical model. Under this medical model, health services are conceived only in terms of hospitals, dispensaries, doctors, and nurses and not in terms of other factors such as food, housing, and water which may affect health and well-being. In times of war more medical personnel, especially surgeons, are hired and medical equipment is purchased with war victims in mind. Thus in war time health policies of African countries become narrow and unidimensional, focusing as it were, on soldiers and perhaps a few people in the privileged class. In these circumstances, rural and urban poor are ignored or at best given only skeletal services. Countries such as Chad and Ethiopia which have been involved in political conflicts for many years may not want to focus their health policies on rural and urban people but rather on war victims. The resources voted for health in times of war are small and only enough primarily to meet the needs of soldiers. It is not possible, therefore, for health policy to concurrently embark on heavy defense spending and a popular health care system.

The impact of violence on health policy is perhaps best demonstrated in the case of the Nigerian civil war of 1967-1970. During the war, health programs started earlier were abandoned and others destroyed. Hospitals, medical equipment, and a medical

174

school were destroyed. The Enugu medical school and the University of Nigeria at Nsukka were destroyed, halting the training of medical personnel for at least three years. Physicians, nurses, and other health personnel lost their lives while many hospitals not destroyed were mobilized for wounded soldiers. The war atmosphere prevented the development of commerce, industry, and farming. No wonder Nigeria was affected by famine both during and after the civil war. The magnitude of physical and psychological destruction was so great that it affected public policy and especially health policy.

After the civil war ended in 1970, the then head of state, General Gowon, embarked on a program of reconciliation and reconstruction. The implication of the reconstruction on health policy was obvious. The renovation of hospitals and clinics destroyed during the war became the focus during the years 1970-1975. Had there not been a war, health policy during the period would have been directed perhaps to rural health care. But as a result of the war, it was not until 1975 after reconstruction was completed that a new health policy was initiated. This time health policy shifted from the predominantly curative one of the civil war to the introduction of Basic Health Services Scheme. In the educational sector, universal primary education (UPE) was introduced. Both programs targeted the rural and urban poor. One would not be wrong to suggest that these policies would have been introduced earlier had resources not been diverted to the war.

The Nigerian example is applicable to many other African countries engaged in political conflicts. In war, such countries lack the stability to think of health policies that would encourage immunization, health education, oral rehydration therapy, child and welfare clinics, and the training of public health workers.

To be sure, the effect of violence on health policy is not limited to civil war. The ten violent religious riots which occurred in Nigeria between May 1980 and March 1987 destroyed several hospitals, clinics, drug stores, hotels, cars, schools, and churches which the government had to renovate. It also had to bear the cost of compensating victims. This kind of violence affects health policy in the sense that resources voted for health education, child welfare, and immunization are again shifted to hospitals to provide for victims or to replace destroyed hospitals. Thus the growth of

175

public health policy is disallowed while curative medicine continues to thrive.

The incessant incidents of violence and political conflict have contributed to the consolidation of curative health policies in Africa. Victims of war or riots, policy makers argue, cannot be treated with primary health care, but in hospitals. On the other hand, policy makers need to understand that infectious diseases, common killers in Africa, cannot be prevented by the building of new hospitals but rather with a comprehensive public health policy that emphasizes good housing, water, food, and a clean environment.

Health Policies and Refugees

Refugee problems are not new to Africa, nonetheless their upsurge and consistency has been disturbing. The number of refugees in Africa has doubled every five years since the 1960s. In 1965, for example, the estimated refugee population of Africa was half a million people, in 1970 one million, in 1975 two million, in 1978 four million. By the end of 1980, the number reached five million.[18] This latter figure is more than the total population of more than the ten smallest African states.[19] By 1984, it was stated that half of the then ten million of the world's refugee population were living in Africa and under distressing circumstances.

The seriousness of the refugee problem in Africa arises from the fact that every instance of protracted violence and conflict in Africa has produced refugee victims. In 1957, the first African political refugees numbering 200,000 fled from Algeria into Morocco and Tunisia as a result of the Algerian war of independence with France. In 1961, about 151,000 Angolan refugees fled into Zaire as a result of the beginning of the war of liberation with Portugal. This figure grew higher between 1961 and 1977, reaching 400,000 by 1970. By 1972, the influx of Burundi refugees into Tanzania and Zaire had reached between 25,000 and 28,000 respectively. In 1979, about 200,000 Zimbabwean refugees were settled all over Africa, especially in the frontline states. Other surveys show that since 1965, more than 250,000 Chadians have fled their territory into the Cameroon, the Central African Republic, and Nigeria to avoid the scourge of war. By 1981, there were 1.5 million refugees living in Somalia alone; 490,000 in

176

Sudan, and 400,000 in Zaire. Other countries which reported more than 100,000 refugees in their territory were Cameroon (266,000), Burundi (234,000), Tanzania (140,000), Uganda (112,400), and Nigeria (110,000). There are also thousands of political refugees from South Africa living in the frontline states.

Refugees suffer from death, disease, and hunger. The rate of crude mortality of Eritrean and Tigrayan refugees in Sudan, for instance, was estimated at 105 per thousand while malnutrition was found to be 52 percent for children under five with less than 80 percent weight per standard height. The occurrence of infectious diseases such as malaria, yellow fever, and typhoid also have been reported in the refugee camps in Africa.[20] The problem of infectious diseases is compounded by the nature of housing available for refugees. Many homes are make-shift and people have problems obtaining water. A large percentage of African refugees are housed in UN refugee camps. However, housing is usually smaller than the population of refugees to be accommodated. The condition is even worse in camps run by national African governments, as they experience constant shortages of food, water, and clothing. On the average refugee camps run by UN and religious groups are better than public camps under the responsibility of African governments.

The living and health conditions of refugees vary widely on the basis of camps where they are accommodated. There may be improvements in the health and living conditions of some camps such as Eritrean and Tigrayan refugees in Sudan, but not in those of Zambia and Angola.[21]

Health issues such as infectious diseases, stress, poor health care, poor sanitation, lack of water, and insufficient food immediately begin to develop as refugees embark on the journey outside their homes. Refugees that spontaneously move across international borders or go far away from their homes are most often accommodated in temporary houses and makeshift huts. From there they begin immediately to face emergency programs of feeding and health. Where large numbers have been involved, the camps often have been squalid and the people malnourished with high mortality rates of 110 per thousand or more in some camps. Hanne Christensen in her study of refugee resettlement in Africa found a high incidence of disease and death in refugee camps in Zambia, Sudan, and Angola in different times of conflict.[22] T. F.

Detts has shown that most refugee camps in Africa have the tendency of dumping large numbers of newly arrived refugees on existing settlement sites without change in existing food supply and health care facilities.[23]

Under such camp conditions, health problems become rampant. These include communicable diseases, anaemia, and nutritional deficiencies (notably kwasiokor), septic abortion, complication of pregnancies, prenatal deaths, and suicide. Degenerative diseases such as peptic ulcers, nephrosis, and diabetes as well as bronchitis and appendicitis also tend to increase under camp pressure and anxiety. Though the quality of statistical data regarding the health of refugees in Africa is less than impeccable, casual observations in most camps by some medical doctors, especially those who were involved in the refugee camps in Biafra during Nigeria's civil war, point to the high concentration among refugee children of such diseases as pneumonia, tuberculosis, diphtheria, smallpox, meningitis, whooping cough, and measles.

Medically, the severe malnutrition which persists in most African refugee camps such as those in Zambia and Sudan may result in clinical complications either in the long or short run. Persistent diarrhea which also occurs in most forms as well as kwasiokor result in liver enlargement and oedema. There is neurological involvement in pellagra and beriberi, bone malformation in acute cases of rickets which are also common, and blindness in the final state of vitamin A deficiency common in refugee children. All these health problems may not be uncommon, but when they result from violence and conflict, they impose serious strains on the health facilities of host countries. This certainly affects health care services and health care programming of the concerned areas. Refugees also strain the health resources of host countries especially in cases where international agencies such as UNICEF do not assist and where the health resources of the best countries are already inadequate. According to Ibrahim Dagash of the OAU Information Division the refugee camps in the Horn of Africa

> are living examples of waste, misery and homelessness. The only way to identify them is that they are refugees for whom only God, the Almighty, knows what the future holds . . . How those refugees manage to live in

178

their present camps under such conditions of poverty, with their children not knowing where to go is a miracle.[24]

If African refugees have strained social infrastructures (notably health) of the host countries, how has this problem been dealt with? Integration or voluntary repatriation of refugees have been regarded as the best solutions. However, those options require the fulfillment of two prerequisites:

1.   There must be the political will by the host state to remedy the plight of refugees in the short run before repatriation, and this must involve taking responsibility for health care of refugees

2.   Integration must demand the reprogramming and maintenance of existing social infrastructures such as health facilities, if refugees are to receive the same quality of medical attention as citizens or residents of their area of refuge. This of course depends on the economic strength of a country to provide health services to all citizens as well as refugees to be integrated

Whether the host countries adopt a policy of voluntary repatriation of refugees or integration, increased social spending in the area of health must accompany budgetary policies of states if refugees' welfare is to be affected. Where the countries of asylum are visibly poor or facing economic readjustments as most African states do, constant mobility of refugees across borders can no longer be ignored as isolated questions in social policies of African states, especially in the area of health, in the face of declining international concern for African refugees.

At the end of the 1980s, funds from external donors to assist host countries cope with social consequences of refugees have been drying up. The reasons for donors' weariness over African refugee problems include the following:

1.   Many donors now believe that some African countries see refugee situations as some kind of industry through which money can be obtained for other pressing social services in their states. This accusation came from the realization that donations to Ethiopian refugees were diverted to other projects

179

2.   Donors also have become skeptical about unrealistic projects submitted by host countries for refugee asylum, in which the basis of improving refugee welfare are not clearly reflected in existing social policies. Some USA and Canadian donors prefer to participate in distributing their donations to refugees so as to forestall any diversion as was the case in the wake of the Ethiopian hunger crisis of 1985

3.   Many donors are concerned that African countries are doing very little to address the political issues that in the first place led to refugees in Africa.[25]

What the views presented here vividly point to is that refugee problems in fact do hinder the health policies of African states in a way that makes the problem a regional issue. An attempt to further understand African refugee problems and how they affect the health policies of African states therefore must be premised on a regional policy focusing on the management of African conflicts and attempts to minimize violence. It is also necessary to prevent the diversion of funds for social programs into security matters. Addressing the root of this problem must not be ignored by African states. As Jake Miller pathetically put the refugee problem:

> No sound is more distressing than the plea of the homeless. Their cry expresses the plea of hunger, thirst and disease, and denotes the fear of death, insecurity and repression. The cry is not pretence, but a reflection of grim reality. It is an expression of tragedy occurring daily through the world, but especially in Africa where one out of every two refugees resides.[26]

Where African conflicts do not directly cause refugee problems, they make the health problem associated with it more difficult to handle. Disease and hunger emerging in Ethiopia, Mozambique, and Uganda are not isolated from the series of protracted conflicts that have occurred in these countries since the 1970s. The starvation that rocked Ethiopia in 1984-1985 can be explained partly by the pressure of refugees produced by the disastrous Ogaden wars. This situation was merely worsened by the scourge of natural disaster. In 1987 an outbreak of cholera was reported in Uganda. Experts relate the health developments in

Uganda to the debilitating condition of protracted conflict in the country and the decaying social services. Mozambique has also been experiencing starvation in which about three million people were affected in 1987. South Africa's constant destabilization of Mozambique has contributed in no small measure to the deteriorating social condition in that country. The inability to find solutions to violence and conflict in Africa means that Africa may continue to endanger the health status of its inhabitants.

Summary

In this chapter, we have tried to chart the direct causal relationship between Africa's many cases of violence and conflict on one hand and health care policies of African states on the other. Specifically, we have examined the impact of African conflict and violence on military expenditure and how these relate to health care. We posit that damages resulting from wars and other violence in Africa affect long-term health programs in African states.

The reduction in the incidence of war refugees in Africa may lead to the improvement of health care services in host and affected states as health policies would be based on the nature of health problems rather than on the need of war victims. We conclude that no state, however humane or prepared, can effectively take care of the health demands of its citizens in the wake of political insecurity, violence, and conflicts. It will be even more difficult when national resources are heavily skewed in favor of defence expenditure.

181

NOTES

1. World Health Organization, *The Work of WHO 1982-1983: The Biennial Report of the Director General to WHO Assembly and the UN* (Geneva: World Health Organization, 1984).
2. Leo O. Ogba, *Emerging Pattern of Conflict Management in Africa: The Role of Nigeria 1960-1983*, Ph.D. diss., University of Toronto, 1986.
3. Pat McGowan and Thomas H. Johnson, "African Military Coup d'Etat and Underdevelopment: A Quantitative Historical Analysis," *Journal of Modern African Studies* 28 (1984): 633-66.
4. *The Military Balance* published by the Institute of Strategic Studies, London, 1980.
5. U.S. Department of State, "African Refugees," *GIST* (April 1981).
6. "1985 Budget Allocations," *West Africa* March 11, 1985.
7. Morris Davis, *Civil War and the Politics of International Relief: Africa, South Asia and the Caribbean* (New York: Praeger, 1975), 8-23.
8. Dennis A. Ityavyar, *The Development of Health Services in Nigeria 1960-1985*, Ph.D. diss., University of Toronto, 1985, p. 137.
9. *Military Balance 1984-1985* (London: International Institute of Strategic Studies, 1984), pp. 40-141.
10. "The Voice of America," *Africa News*, 19th February 1987.
11. Ibid., and Julie Cliff, et al., "Mozambique Health Holding the Line," *Review of African Political Economy* 36 (1986): 7-23.
12. Academic Staff Union of Universities, *The Killings of ABU*, Zaria Academic Staff Union, 1986.
13. S. O. Alubo, "State Violence and Health in Nigeria," mimeographed, 1987.

14. Organization of African Unity, The Council of Ministers, 14th Ordinary Session Resolution C14/1239 (XL) Addis Ababa, 1984.
15. Godfrey Gunati-Ileke, *Inter-Sectoral Linkages and Health Development*, WHO offset Pub. No. 83, 1984, pp. 7-9.
16. Olof Palme et al., "Military Spending; the Economic and Social Consequences," *Challenge* September/October 1982, p. 15.
17. The World Bank, *Accelerated Development in Sub-Saharan Africa: An Agenda for Action* (Washington: World Bank, 1983), p. 67.
18. Organization of African Unity, The Council of Ministers, *Creating Contemporary Fund for Refugees* (Addis Ababa, 1984).
19. C. J. Bakwasegha, "Development Options and the African Refugee Problems," *The African Refugee* 5 (1984): 8.
20. The authors acknowledge here information on social and health conditions of refugees as provided by anonymous reviews who drew from the work of Roger Brown, a physician who worked with UN refugee camps.
21. *The Africa Refugee* 3/4 (1983): 11.
22. Hanne Christensen, *The Problem of Refugee Settlement in Africa* (Geneva: Geneva International University Exchange Fund, 1978), p. 7.
23. T. F. Retts, "Evaluation and Promotion of Integrated Rural Development: Approach to Refugee problems in Africa," *Africa Today* 31 (1984): 20.
24. *The African Refugee* 5 (June 1984/85): 3.
25. Ibid.
26. Jake Miller, "The Homeless of Africa," *Africa Today* 37 (1989): 32.

10

HEALTH INEQUALITIES IN AFRICA

Tola Olu Pearce

Introduction

In this chapter, an attempt will be made to understand the ways in which social relationships and social organizations contribute significantly to health inequalities. Health and ill-health have been described as social products in so far as they can be viewed as expressions of patterns of interaction, macro and micro-level relationships, and people's ability to rally resources to combat an onslaught.[1] The Western biomedical model which perceives disease as random attacks from nature or largely initiated from the biological and physical spheres of life is increasingly believed to be superficial in its approach to disease. One well-known argument is that physicians alleviate health problems only to recycle the patient back to the same social environment in which he or she is likely to develop the same malady. Within a given society, certain roles, positions, and experiences expose people to certain types of diseases. In a study of society and social change, Abrams argued that our explanation of occurrences must develop from an understanding of the paradox of social life.[2] This paradox is that men's activities create phenomena (institutions, objects, meanings, emotions) which then confront the actors to produce important changes in the subjects themselves. There is a perpetual interaction between subjects and the objects which they create. The development of disease in human populations should not be seen as escaping this interaction. Thus, as values, beliefs, attitudes, and power relations are translated into social activity and networks, various groups within society tend to have differential access to those factors which are now believed to affect health. These

184

include food, income, education, leisure time, social services information, medical services, decision-making bodies, and social/emotional support. For instance, disadvantaged groups in society have less access to the most advanced or prestigious medical services within any historical period than advantaged groups.[3] In addition, the social definition of an abnormality such as disease, crime, laziness, or sin, and its acceptance as worthy of medical attention can affect its spread and outcome within a particular segment of the population.[4] Religious, political, and economic ideologies play an important role in forming definitions. In creating institutions and customs, people also manipulate the physical and biological dimensions of nature and thus affect the prevalence of disease in different subgroups. For example, it can be argued that child birth and its attendant hazards occur only for the female sex and the new offspring. Nevertheless, the burden of disease and death born by this group is largely influenced by custom, technology, beliefs about motherhood, labor needs, and so forth. Thus in agricultural societies with simple technology where labor needs are high and where women are encouraged to produce as many children as possible, the female population will have a greater exposure to the possibility of maternal deaths than in a society where high fertility is seen as obstructing women's economic activities.[5]

Another point of emphasis arising from the work of Abrams and Elias is the view that a person's position in a network of relationships is what defines him.[6] He is never merely an "individual" in an abstract sense, but part of a process or network in which there are consequences for his position. Thus changes in his health status are the outcome of both his position in the matrix and his reaction to this position. Therefore to write that persons are workers in a capitalist system or peasants in a feudal system is to assume that they are embedded in well-defined relationships.[7] It is then necessary to ferret out the (health) consequences of these relationships. The data presented here will be discussed under the three well-known periods in African history: the precolonial, colonial, and post-colonial.

The Precolonial Era

Although less is known about the prevalence and distribution of disease in precolonial Africa than about the two periods which followed, certain observations can be made. First, from the Iron Age to the 1800s epidemics were experienced in waves over all regions within the continent. This is not to suggest that Africa was exceptionally burdened in comparison to the other continents. From ancient times throughout the Middle Ages to the nineteenth century, numerous epidemics also broke out across Europe, the Orient, and the Americas. These included the Black Death, St. Vitus Dance, syphilis, typhus, typhoid fever, smallpox, bacillary dysentery, the Picardy sweat, and cholera.[8] Zinsser's vivid account of the waves of epidemics which followed wars, explorations, famine, the displacement of populations, changes in authority structures, and recurrent impoverishment in Europe reveals the horrendous experience of that continent.[9] Africa's health problems therefore were far from exceptional.

Second, even though local communities were increasingly being opened up for trade and exploration by Arabs and Europeans after the sixteenth century, societies maintained substantial control over their socioeconomic environment until the colonial period. This, together with the levels of immunity against local diseases, is believed to have been a major factor in disease control in the African interior.[10] Finally, the great diversity in the structure of settlements over Africa must be appreciated. From the early Iron Age down to the nineteenth century, kingdoms rose and fell, centralized governments developed and social inequalities crystallized in some regions (Ethiopia, Uganda, and in Ghana among the Asante). However, other settlements remained small, homogenous and relatively egalitarian (the Tonga and Igbo). Also, some communities underwent significant modifications in the structure of male/female relationships and the status of women (for example in Zanzibar). Such diversity would preclude the development of a single or composite configuration of the distribution of disease in precolonial populations. Nonetheless, our knowledge about the characteristics of some of the diseases which appeared at the time and about the structures of communities, allow tentative comments.

186

In any region or community, a disease can either be seen as long standing or new. In addition, it may be communicable or noncommunicable. Long standing/local communicable diseases such as sleeping sickness, certain types of malaria, yellow fever, intestinal and skin problems originated in Africa or had been around for centuries. Local populations had developed patterns of immunity to these diseases. "Disease environments" arising from local histories and geographical factors influenced each community's pattern of immunity. Curtin has hypothesized that because of the relative isolation of communities in the African interior, "disease environments would have been more diverse than those of Europe."[11] Thus within the numerous disease environments, distribution patterns would have been influenced by ongoing social relationships or structures. The new or alien diseases spread across the continent in the wake of trade and exploration occurring largely since the sixteenth century. Although these may have had either African or non-African origin, their effect on the new non-immunized community was likely to be the same. Those of non-African origin included tuberculosis, measles, smallpox, and cholera. In the second category fall diseases such as malaria which was familiar to West Africa but were transplanted to other places such as Ruanda as the continent was opened up.[12] Sleeping sickness was another case in point, as can be deduced from the following statement: "When Stanley crashed through the jungle from the Congo to Uganda to rescue Emin Pasha, sleeping sickness carried by Palpalis must have followed him."[13] Mckelvey had noticed that the spread of sleeping sickness followed Stanley's tracks. Finally, increased interregional movements brought local populations in contact with new strains of long-standing diseases against which they were not yet protected.[14]

Examples of noncommunicable health problems include malnutrition, various mental disorders, and problems associated with female circumcision. Such health disorders are related to indigenous customs and exposure to geographical hazards. Any transformations within the system may result in the disappearance of old disorders and/or the development of new ones. Thus when the Wapogoro of Southeastern Tanzania retreated to a restricted landmass as a result of interethnic wars in the nineteenth century, their semi-nomadic life changed to a sedentary one on less fertile soil. Regular famine and nutritional deficiencies appear to have contributed to the development of a disorder of the nervous system known as *kifafa* in that area.[15]

Although the disparity in living conditions between the rich and the poor in precolonial societies generally did not reach the proportions experienced in Europe during the same period, they became appreciable within some communities.[16] For instance, trade produced significant differences in wealth in the empires along the West coast and the Sudan. In some places, the gap between the rulers and the ruled, slaves and landlords or between different castes were reinforced by legal rights and exploitative production relationships. Restricted access to many items, particularly food, affected the health of members of the lower strata. Among the Bulosi of the upper Zambezi, a large portion of the population were slaves who had very limited rights. Their masters' lands had to be cultivated, various other duties performed, and harsh treatment was normal. They were allocated the poorest soils for their own needs, debarred from eating the more prestigious foods and from using the more durable materials for housing. Again, travelling freemen could help themselves to the harvest of slaves.[17] Maquet discussed the exploitative relationship between the Tutsi and Butu in Ruanda and argued that the diet of the latter was inadequate for his physical welfare.[18] In addition, the more leisurely existence of the Tutsi allowed the development of a subculture in which more hygienic practices could be adhered to them among the Rutu.

Such social arrangements usually are marked by noticeable differences in the distribution of both communicable and non-communicable diseases. With respect to the long-standing or local diseases, there is evidence that the disadvantaged groups carried a heavier burden. Tedlie, writing in 1819, reported that among the Asante diseases such as yaws, the itch (psora), and ringworm were much more common among slaves and the poorer classes than the upper groups.[19] This he attributed to their poorer diet, bad living conditions, and overwork. The best medical attention was also reserved for the rich.[20]

Among the Bulosi mentioned earlier, hunger and starvation were common occurrences in the slave population. All this is not to suggest that the presence of slaves or lower strata in a society always indicated serious differences in the social conditions of groups. The situation depended on the "entitlement relationships" present in the society.[21] Where slaves were allowed to obtain their freedom, become members of the kingroup, and marry free women (Yoruba, pre-nineteenth century Kereba) they "lived usually as well as their masters. . . . Their social standing was, for the most part, not much inferior to that of others."[22] Likewise, the Tenne had developed a system in which resources were constantly being redistributed to the lower strata so that wide social disparities were unable to develop.[23]

A few diseases were more prevalent among the richer classes. In Mali, during the fourteenth century, sleeping sickness is believed to have been more common among the privileged groups.[24] Perhaps one can suggest that the dependence of the tsetse fly on horses and other animals exposed those groups who could afford or had the rights to such animals to sleeping sickness.

The recurrent epidemics of alien diseases recorded at this time are said to have been stimulated by trade, travel, warfare, and drought. Smallpox for example became frequent after 1500 in West Africa, the Sudan, Angola, Ethiopia, and East Africa. Similarly sand fly fever, the plague, some venereal diseases, and tuberculosis disturbed many communities decade after decade. The actual experience of communities no doubt depended on a number of factors. First, communities were differentially exposed to these epidemics. Proximity to trade routes and commercial centers was important. Those along trade routes often had epidemics every three to five years compared to from seven to ten years for those further away, while a distant region would have few incidences.[25] Second, population concentration and the growth of cities was also more conducive to raging epidemics than thinly populated regions. Timbuktu was believed to have lost about half of its population during the epidemics and famines of the early eighteenth century. Third, initial exposure was likely to have resulted in the maturation of the population because of the absence of immunity. This can be deduced from the behavior of new infections which had disturbed Europe when medical science was less capable of protecting the rich.[26] After the first epidemic, periodic outbreaks occurred when conditions permitted. Smallpox, for example, usually reappeared during droughts, famines, and periods of political disorganization when people lost access to food, shelter, and other resources (such as across West Africa during the seventeenth and eighteenth centuries). Depending on the disease and its mode of transmission,

189

in subsequent outbreaks the pattern of infection and case fatality rate would begin to approximate those of the long standing diseases if advantaged groups were able to command resources for host resistance (for example, inoculation, isolation, and nutrition).

In sum, it can be said that from the sixteenth century, Africa was disturbed by waves of new diseases which established themselves alongside the local ones. Their initial effect is believed to have been devastating to the non-immunized populations. Local or long standing diseases already showed a pattern in which prevalence was more for the lower strata in those communities where important socioeconomic inequalities had arisen. Malnutrition, starvation, and communicable diseases such as malaria, sleeping sickness, and yaws were the common health problems at this time. In this respect, Africa did not differ from the other continents in the pattern of diseases.

The Colonial Era

During the period which lasted roughly from the late nineteenth century to the 1960s, much of Africa was under political domination and all of it was increasingly penetrated by capitalism. Throughout this period there were numerous campaigns against specific diseases. A few such as those against yaws and smallpox were successful. This notwithstanding, the colonial period was marked by increased deterioration in the health of large segments of the African population. Sizable discrepancies developed between the health status of the average European and African citizen. For instance, life expectancy at birth for 1950-1955 was below 50 years in all the regions of Africa. It was lowest in Western Africa (32.0 years) and highest in Southern Africa (43.2 years).[27] For England and Wales, the 1950-1952 figures for males and females were 66.4 years and 71.5 years respectively.[28] In France, between 1952 and 1956 on the average males could expect to live 65 years and females 71 years.[29] The figures for Africa closely resembled those of Europe in the mid-nineteenth century. For example in France the figures were 39 years for males and 40 for females by 1861-1865. In 1841 males had a life expectancy of 40.2 years and females 42.2 years for England and Wales. Towards the end of the colonial period, in 1960, the infant mortality and crude death rates tell the same story. For example, while Kenya and Senegal had infant mortality rates of 112 and 178 per 1,000, those of Britain and Western Germany were 23 and 34 per 1,000 respectively.[30] Communicable diseases were brought under control in the West, but in Africa they were still the major health problem along with nutritional diseases. Thus diseases such as malaria, gastroenteritis, pneumonia, filariasis, sleeping sickness, schistosomiasis, and measles as well as malnutrition even gained ground in many places.

The harsh picture generally presented for the continent must be understood as one dimension of the consequences of colonization. Political domination and the loss of control over their affairs led to new disruptions in community life. The disruptions hitherto experienced by the slave trade and other commercial ventures were limited compared to the new situation. Agricultural and economic policies were designed by the various colonial administrations to make the colonies self-supporting, to generate surplus for developing the colonizing nation, to help finance the world wars, and to pay off war debts. These altered indigenous production patterns, living arrangements and methods of coping with unforeseen disasters. The demand for cash crops such as groundnut, coffee, cocoa, cotton, wine, and rubber led to the growth of plantations, private ownership of land, neglect of food crops, and the expansion of production into less fertile areas or tsetse fly infested zones. Often, villages which did not produce the required goods were punished.[31] Forced labor was common throughout the continent as were monetary taxes, appropriation of land, and the opening up of mines.[32]

As many scholars have pointed out, the consequences were disastrous. For example, Shenton and Watts have argued that when indigenous methods of communal farming as well as grain taxation and storage were interrupted by British policies in Northern Nigeria, communities lost their ability to feed themselves adequately, organize relief in the face of droughts, and store grains for the future.[33] Whenever farmers were not allowed to decide, according to their own knowledge of the area, where crops were to be planted, herds to be grazed or even their own habitat, areas infested by the tsetse fly increased as a result of ecological disruptions. In Malawi, thirty years of colonization resulted in the doubling of the area occupied by the fly. This pattern of change was repeated across the continent.[34] Both the introduction of

191

taxes and forced labor induced the movement of men from their farms to areas of wage employment in the cities, mines, and plantations. The consequences of this migration were felt in both the labor supplying rural areas and the new settlements. In the former, women, children, and the elderly with minimal resources were left to produce crops on smaller farms.[35] Migration weakened family ties and support systems considerably, while the migrants' low wages meant that the cost of reproducing their labor was largely borne by families in the rural areas.[36] In the urban centers, mining or railway camps and plantations, working conditions and living standards were far below what would sustain good health.[37]

Besides this loss of control over the economic aspects of life, Feierman draws our attention to the fact that changes in the power base of the indigenous practitioners themselves had far reaching effects on their ability to control health.[38] In the precolonial days, healers and priests were usually part of the power structure. An important dimension of their ability to maintain health levels in communities was derived from their public authority. Thus in conjunction with other leaders they directed public activities such as the movement of villagers away from hazardous locations, the building of irrigation projects, the disposal of waste, or control of deviant behavior. Their subsequent loss of access to the arena where issues affecting health were debated relegated them to the limited area of clinical care or the private encounter. One should note that this development becomes significant in a situation where the newly imported medical system was unable effectively to cover most of the colony. In addition to this, both the missionaries and the Western medical practitioners attacked indigenous systems which were then faced with the problem of legitimacy. Both financial and human resources within the colonies were made available to the Western medical system for its development. Thus having lost its legal footing, indigenous medicine was unable to command manpower and finances for research and expansion as did the Western approach to healing.

Another important way in which colonization affected health was through the changes brought about in the stratification systems of the different nations. In some instances, a rural elite developed where the community had been relatively egalitarian. Dixon-Fyle discussed how a stratum of wealthy farmers developed among the Tonga of Zambia after the introduction of wage economy, the plough, and the private ownership of land.[39] By 1945, about 15 percent of the population had become large cultivators hiring the labor of others. In other areas (Sierra Leone, the former Gold Coast, Sudan, and Burundi) the policy of indirect rule of colonial administrations pitted real or imagined ruling classes against the peasantry. Whether in Uganda or Northern Nigeria rulers and leaders were incorporated into the new administration to which they were now accountable.[40] Their position was that of middlemen used to maintain law and order, collect taxes, and organize the execution of government projects. While performing their duties they were also able to extract benefits for themselves in terms of extra levies, bribes and forced labor from the peasants and social amenities from the administration. The point to be emphasized here is that the former rights and duties which had existed in the old hierarchical relationships were changed fundamentally. The result was that the local farmers lost their leaders for duties performed. Continuous increases in taxation, the growing food needs of the cities, and rising cost of the new, imported goods all assisted in shifting the position of the peasantry from one which could command supplies of goods for its needs (either by ownership, purchasing, or recognized rights) to one which lost access to sufficient supplies. In addition, as impoverished sections of the nation they could not demand from the authorities other health-giving amenities.

Notwithstanding the nuances in the precolonial stratification structures or the fact that there were several colonizing powers, a small nucleus of new elites began to appear throughout the continent. This comprised those groups who were able to take advantage of administrative policies and activities. The siting of commercial, administrative, and mining centers along with schools and transportation routes presented opportunities to a few. Often the opportunities for education and employment in white collar jobs were greater for some ethnic groups than others because of the geographical location of colonial activities or the conscious selection of certain groups as middlemen.[41] Thus Bakwesegba narrated how Buganda became a "favored area" where most of the good schools and industries were built. "By Independence Day in 1962, 50 percent of the Ugandan elite and three-quarters of the civil service personnel were Buganda."[42] Similar imbalances were

193

created in other countries such as Sierra Leone, Nigeria, Kenya, and the Sudan. In addition, some precolonial ruling classes and merchant capitalists were able to secure education and skilled jobs for their families, as were descendants of freed slaves and those in close contact with missionary work. Besides the colonial rulers, these groups were the next beneficiaries of the agricultural and commercial surplus produced during the colonial period. They therefore had better access to adequate housing, water, medical facilities, and food compared to the peasants and the unskilled wage earners.

In a book entitled *A World of Differentials*, Abdin and associates detail the process by which a wide gap was created between the salaries and living standards of the educated elite and the rest of the African urban community. In the British territories, for example, a unified civil service was structured after the mid-1940s. Africans were now allowed into the senior service cadre, and they received substantial salaries to help run the bureaucratic system that had been developed. The salary differential in Nigeria for five years reveal growing discrepancies as one moves from the clerical staff to the top civil servants (Table 1). At the time of independence in 1960, the degree of inequality was still high. While the bottom 40 percent received about 19 percent of the wage bill, the top 10 percent received about 43 percent of it.[43]

Migrant workers in the mines, factories, plantation, and construction firms formed another segment of the emerging stratification. In 1954 the Carpenter Committee on African wages in Kenya reported that half of the workers in private industry "were receiving wages insufficient to provide for the basic needs of a single man, let alone a man with his wife and children." Housing became a perennial problem and most workers were forced to find lodgings in the shantytown areas. Thus in 1962, 70 percent of the African households in Nairobi lived in one-room homes. Forty-nine percent of the houses in the city had three or more persons per room.[44] Some of the manual workers on the plantations and estates were among the most wretched in society. Vail and White's descriptions of the condition of plantation workers in Mozambique bear this out. Similar accounts can be found however for workers in the former Congo, in Angola, and in Southern Africa. In Mozambique, Portugal's persistent drive for high cotton and sugar production encouraged many companies to institute stringent work demands in their estates. In 1940, one company insisted that "every person, including the children irrespective of age, was to have half a hectare of land cleared by November, and another half a hectare cleared by December; that the cotton seed was to be planted before any food crops; and that anyone who failed to comply would be sent to the administration for punishment."[45] Punishment included beatings, locking babies up in containers, imprisonment, and sexual assault. As in other countries, the labor was often initially obtained through raids on villages.

Table 1

NIGERIA: RATIO OF TOP SALARY IN EACH BRANCH
TO BOTTOM SUBORDINATE SALARY

Year	Clerical	Technical and Executive	Professional and Administrative[1]	Superscale
1945	26.4	45.0	55.5	150.0
1950	13.1	17.5	23.8	48.2
1953	11.8	19.5	23.4	58.5
1955	8.0	15.3	15.3	40.0
1960	7.9	15.1	15.1	37.1

[1]Excluding medical extension

Source: Abdin, A., et al. *A World of Differentials*, p. 55.

The conclusion to be drawn from the above discussion is that apart from an overall increase in the volume of disease experienced during the colonial period, there were deepening health inequalities. The higher socioeconomic status of non-African populations coupled with their greater access to the benefits of Western medicine allowed them to enjoy better health than the blacks as revealed by the data on three groups in Nairobi (Table 2).

Table 2

INFANT MORTALITY RATES PER 1,000 LIVE BIRTHS,
NAIROBI 1955-1959

Population Group	1955	1956	1957	1958	1959
European	18.0	19.9	28.6	31.7	25.7
Asian	48.0	49.8	46.2	38.9	44.5
African	111.0	130.5	98.3	89.8	103.8

Source: Fendall, N. *Public Health Reports* 78/7: 1968, p. 581.

Among Africans there were health status differentials along a number of dimensions. These consisted of regional, urban/rural, and class. Thus advantaged geopolitical regions recorded more favorable health statistics than depressed or neglected zones.[46] In rural Gambia for example, Gamble discovered in the late 1940s that while the infant mortality rate was 525 per 1,000 in a very poor village, it was 333 on one where a development project had been established and 165 in a prosperous (agricultural) village.[47] Similarly, data from Sierra Leone in the 1930s reveal that still births were higher for women in the protectorate than the colony (Freetown and Kissy Division). In the protectorate a woman could expect to have 0.45 still births from a total of 4.91 births. In the colony, a woman had an average 0.16 still births of 4.16 births.[48] Sometimes medical services were located near European enterprises to improve the health of the labor force. In the Ivory Coast Lasker discovered that during the depression new hospitals and maternity centers were most likely to be built where the French had plantations.[49] After 1945, medicine was also used as a political weapon. Those geopolitical regions in which there was growing opposition to the French presence received fewer facilities.

Turning now to urban/rural trends, it can be said that rural dwellers suffered more although there were problem areas within the cities too. Rural famine and malnutrition became more persistent as peasants struggled to feed the new cities, neglected food crops for cash crops, and grew less nutritious, high yielding plants such as cassava. Such problems were reported all over West Africa, from Senegal to the Sudan, and across to Ethiopia, as well

196

as East Africa.[50] Epidemics such as influenza and meningitis in Northern Nigeria during the early 1920s took a very heavy toll among the hungry peasants.[51] Although only a few urban/rural comparisons exist for this period, the standard health indicators reveal higher death rates in the rural areas. Thus in 1955 the infant mortality rate in Lagos, a city in the southwestern region of Nigeria, was 82 per 1,000 live births. For villages in the same region, Calletti et al. recorded rates as high as 304. Nicol also found urban (350 per 1,000) and rural (389 per 1,000) differences for the northern region in 1958.[52] Although rural dwellers suffered significantly from many of the communicable diseases, the overcrowding in the poor urban households and shantytown neighborhoods resulted in a higher prevalence of some diseases. Such was the case of tuberculosis. Studies conducted by the World Health Organization in the late 1950s disclosed higher urban rates in many countries within the different regions of Africa.

Even within a single location the economic leverage of certain groups meant better health. Central Lagos, known as the island, grew rapidly and by the 1930s was already known as a high density slum area with few sanitary facilities. When the bubonic plague broke out in 1924, it was confined to the island and part of the mainland adjacent to it (Iddo).[53] The rest of the mainland contained some higher income neighborhoods such as Apapa, Ikeja, parts of Surulere, Ebute-Metta, and Yaba. Social amenities such as modern toilet systems, water supply, refuse removal, and tarred roads were more likely to be found in such locations. The 1955 death rates tell part of the story. On the island the crude death rate was 53.5 per 1,000 but only 5.7 per 1,000 for the mainland. The infant mortality rates were 105.5 and 30.8 per 1,000 respectively.[54]

Migrant workers living in a city or within the special work camps and agricultural estates owned by European companies were a particularly vulnerable segment of the population. For instance, workers were significantly affected by famines and food shortages. This led to sharp rises in the price of food and the workers' meager wages became grossly insufficient. Away from their families and farms, eating patterns changed and the quality of diets suffered. The increased consumption of alcohol became a problem as did venereal diseases due to the growth of prostitution. In Nairobi, for example, there was a male/female ratio of one to eight by the late 1940s. Whenever the price of export crops fell workers lost many of their benefits. Their salaries were reduced, their food rations decreased, and their movements were monitored more closely. Nevertheless, production output was expected to increase to secure continued profit.[55] Migrant workers on the highly controlled company estates and plantations were susceptible to nutritional diseases such as pellagra as a result of vitamin deficient diets. Shortages of protein foods were also quite common.[56] The various groups of migrant workers were a constant source of contamination for their communities of origin. They returned with a variety of infectious diseases such as tuberculosis as well as venereal and helminth diseases.

The colonial period must be remembered as a time when the volume of disease steadily increased on the continent. This resulted from the uprooting of people, disruptions in their pattern of eating and working, new occupational stresses, and alterations in former rights and obligations which had bound people together within their communities. Most changes were enforced without consultation which made adjustment more difficult. Furthermore, inequalities in wealth became more common in country after country as new class structures began to take shape (for example the growth of the urban wage earner, educated elite, and rural proletariat). These changes were expressed in group differences in health conditions. The pattern of diseases had not changed from that of the precolonial period. Thus communicable and nutritional diseases were the main problems. The newer diseases such as cholera, tuberculosis, and venereal diseases had now become endemic. The older problems such as malaria and sleeping sickness had spread over larger areas.

The Post-Colonial Era

After political independence there existed the naive expectation that both economically and in terms of health, conditions would improve significantly. Nevertheless economic independence did not follow for the former colonies and various forms of exploitation have persisted. Processes initiated during the colonial era have matured and one outcome has been the intensification of health inequalities. Another is the continued importance of communicable diseases such as malaria, dysentery, guinea worm,

198

tuberculosis, and measles in the overall pattern of disease. In addition, the problem of malnutrition and nutritional disorders has increased for some groups. If one compared again the health situation of Western and African nations an even wider discrepancy between the two is indicated during this period. For instance, in 1960, the infant mortality rate for Ethiopia at 172 per 1,000 was 7.4 times that of Britain, 6.3 times that of France and 6.6 times that of the USA. However, by 1982, with 122 per 1,000, the Ethiopian rate had risen to 11, 12.2, and 11 times the 1982 rates of Britain, France, and the USA respectively. Such trends have been the norm rather than the exception for most African countries including Nigeria, Mali, Senegal, Zambia, Egypt, and Zimbabwe.[57] The caloric consumption and the life expectancy at birth for a number of Western and African countries merely reinforces what is indicated by the infant mortality rates (Table 3). Although there have been some improvements in Africa, these countries lag far behind the Western ones.

Health remains a major problem because of the low performance of the factors affecting health—per capita income, public health programs, literacy (especially female), and rural development. For example, the GNP per capita for Uganda, Sierra Leone, and Morocco was $230, $390, and $860 respectively in 1982. Only ten of the fifty-three African countries had GNP per capita that were over $1,000. In comparison the figures were $6,840, $9,660, $12,460, and $13,160 for Italy, Britain, Western Germany and the USA.[58] Female literacy remains low. In 1981, the percentage of the eligible female population enrolled in primary schools was below 50 percent in many countries. For example, it was 17 percent in Niger, 20 percent in Mali, 30 percent in Sierra Leone, 33 percent in Ethiopia, and 46 percent in Uganda. However, there was no Western European nation in which it fell below 96 percent.

In most African nations there is a deepening economic crisis; global recession is felt more intensely than in other regions of the world. At the top of the list is the crisis in food production, for although most people are still farmers, there has been a decline in food crop output per head of population in many countries, an exodus from the neglected rural areas, continued diversion of resources into export crop production, and increased importation of food items.[59] Thus foodstuffs such as palm oil, rice, wheat,

199

milk, live animals, fish, and sugar are being imported largely from the industrialized countries. Data for Nigeria reveals that imports of food and live animals as a percentage of total imports doubled in just eight years between 1975 (8 percent) and 1983 (16.3 percent).[60] Many of the items are new and remain difficult to produce locally, thus ensuring future import needs. These food imports coupled with the drain of resources to pay for technological equipment, dividends, royalties, interest, and technical fees ensures that outflow of monies exceeds any inflow gained via investments, loans, and grants.[61] There is therefore a continued paucity of resources to improve the quality of life of African populations.

Table 3

CALORIE CONSUMPTION AND LIFE EXPECTANCY
COMPARISONS FOR SELECTED AFRICAN
AND EUROPEAN NATIONS

Country	% of Daily Caloric Requirement Consumed Per Capita (1981)	Life Expectancy at Birth in 1982	
		Male	Female
Sudan	99	46	49
Guinea	75	37	38
Nigeria	91	48	52
Tanzania	83	51	54
Mozambique	70	49	52
Chad	76	42	45
Britain	132	71	77
France	133	71	79
W. Germany	133	70	77

Source: *World Development Report 1984*. Oxford: World Bank, pp. 262, 264.

The above review of growing inequalities in health between Europeans and Africans however masks the also growing inequalities within Africa. It was suggested earlier that during the precolonial era, economic inequalities were generally greater in

Europe than in Africa. There is evidence that in the post-colonial era this has been reversed. First, the differences between the volume of facilities (such as water, industries, schools, and hospitals) allocated to urban and rural areas has become enormous.[62] In discussing the relationship between national capitals and the surrounding areas Gugber and Flanagan have argued that outside of West African cities one "is stunned by the disparity between the concentration of resources in the capital cities and the neglect that is the fate of much of their hinterlands. . . the hubris of capital cities in West Africa is rooted in the political and social structure of these countries, which tends to appropriate to the capital."[63] In the Ivory Coast, the 1973 doctor/population ratio in Abidjan was 1:3,150. In comparison, the ratio was 1:66,000 in the Western region and 1:64,000 in the North. As Lasker discovered, Abidjan with "one-fifth of the population, consumed 50 percent of the money allocated for medicine and supplies."[64] The urban/rural inequality was said to be basically that of Abidjan versus the rest of the nation.

Similar urban/rural distinctions also have been recorded for Nigeria. Within each state, the state capital and urban centers consume the bulk of the resources. Thus in Ogun State (south-western area) data for 1979 showed that while the doctor/population ration in Abeokuta, the state capital, was 1:11,245 and 1:17,348 in Ijebu Ode, an urban center. It was 1:192,615 in Egbado North and 1:200,861 in Ijebu North, both rural areas. In Abeokuta 72 liters of water were consumed per person per day, but only 3.2 liters and 10.0 liters were available for each person in Egbado North and Ijebu North respectively.[65] Such problems developed elsewhere in Africa. Thirty years after independence in Egypt, 89 percent of the rural population was still without treated drinking water. It depended upon irrigation canals and the Nile River. The four major cities which included Cairo and Alexandria housed 75 percent of the 4,500 doctors available at that time.[66]

Thus the immediate outcome of political independence was increased urban/rural economic disparities. A major cause of this has been the growth in size and power of the elite groups established during the colonial era. Most members of the elite reside in the cities. The planning process developed by the colonialists has been continued by the elite to the present day. Thus both the method of planning and the organization of medical care have remained centralized. Therefore the various disadvantaged groups have minimum access to the inadequate urban and hospital based facilities or the planning committees.[67]

The elite now tend to have a larger share of the national income than their Western counterparts. For example, while the richest 10 percent of Kenya (1972) and Tanzania (1969) had 56.0 percent and 35.6 percent of the nation's income, the same group in Britain (1977) and Sweden (1972) had 23.3 percent and 21.3 percent respectively. In Nigeria the richest 5 percent shared 41 percent of the national income in 1971-1972.[68] Fringe benefits attached to positions and the use of one's status to develop other sources of income greatly augment the economic dominance of the elite. In Kenya, the salaried elite can legitimately run private enterprises, invest in property, or purchase large farms.[69] This is often done covertly elsewhere when the earning of secondary incomes is illegal. The amount accruing from these benefits may actually exceed the base salary for senior civil servants, as in Morocco. However, such benefits only amount to 15 percent of the Moroccan unskilled worker's salary.[70] Finally, where it had been initiated, the class differences within rural populations is now well established. The richer peasants were able to consolidate their advantages and forge business as well as marital connections with the urban elite.[71]

Cliffe and Moorsom's description of rural class formation in Botswana reveals the extent to which the bulk of the peasantry lost access to the means of self-sufficiency over twenty years.[72] Three groups of peasants had developed by 1975. At the top were the rich commercial cattle ranchers. Below them, the middle peasants. These two groups had accrued sizable herds and access to the best farm land. However, 45 percent of the peasants owned no cattle and 66 percent had ten or less. It was believed that at least ten head of cattle were needed for self-sufficiency. About 45 percent of the peasants were estimated to be below the stipulated poverty line. To survive the poorer households became indebted to the richer peasants through arrangements which allowed them to use the latter's animals for draught. Given the increased pressure on the land and the success of the wealthy peasants, any future drought is expected to be devastating, especially for the poorer households which have little or no margin with which to work. While such major disparities within the rural areas may be more

202

common in East and Southern Africa, some differences have also emerged in other regions. In Nigeria for example, Okuneye has argued that "there is abundant evidence suggesting some degree of (rural) income disparity. It is common to identify landlord absenteeism in many rural areas, contrasting sizes of farm lands with an impressive, proportion of landless peasants."[73]

Thus, health differentials continue to follow the pattern that emerged during the colonial era. Again, the major differences are among regions, urban, and rural areas as well as among economic categories. Therefore, areas located towards the north in Nigeria have higher mortality rates than southern regions. The crude mortality rate for Kwara State in 1971 was 25.3 per 1,000. Within the Western State however it was 17.8 and only 9.6 in Lagos. Within regions, urban/rural differences continue to exist. Thus in the Western State the infant mortality rate was 77 per 1,000 in urban centers but 109 in the rural areas. More recent data from one of the states, which was carved out of the old Western State, indicates that differences still exist. In Oyo State the proportion of urban households which lost a child during its first year of life was estimated at 1.7 percent in 1984. In comparison, 3.0 percent of rural households lost an infant. Ekanem and Farooq obtained the same pattern with respect to life expectancy in southwestern Nigeria.[74] In the rural areas, males had an expectancy of 47.2 years and females 47.0 years. However, for urban residents the figures were 50.6 years (male) and 50.8 years (female). The 1969 infant mortality rates as reported by Gregory and Piche for urban and rural comparisons in Burkina Faso, present a similar picture (Table 4).[75]

Finally, there is continued evidence that class membership affects the time of death and types of illnesses experienced by segments of the population. Data on occupational groups in Nigeria show that children of professionals have a higher survival rate at birth than others such as petty traders and agricultural workers. Pearce and Obebiyi also discovered from hospital records in Ibadan that congenital malformations are higher among petty traders than professionals.[76] In addition, the expected negative effects of high parity are more evident among the former group. In South Africa where the benefits of economic privilege by and large accrue to the whites, Asians, Coloured, and Africans in that order, mortality and morbidity rates follow the same trend. Unterhalter has presented mortality rates for Johannesburg between 1910 and 1979. Although crude death and infant mortality rates had fallen for all groups over this period, whites and Asians still fared much better than the Coloureds or Africans. For 1977, the infant mortality rates were given as 16.76 for whites, 18.02 for Asians, 41.38 for Coloureds and 41.73 for Africans.[77] Again, in 1976 the tuberculosis rate for Africans was about 16 times that of the whites. For the Coloureds the rate was 18 times the whites. Similarly, for every white person who had typhoid, 4 Coloured, 5 Asians, and 8 Africans contacted the disease.

Table 4

INFANT MORTALITY RATES AS PERCENTAGE OF
LIVE BIRTHS IN BURKINA FASO (1969)

Ages	Ouagadougou	BoboDioulasso	Rural
15-19	18.1	9.5	27.8
20-24	22.7	17.3	21.9
25-29	24.8	22.6	28.9
30-34	24.2	26.0	31.2

Source: Gregory, J. and Piche, V. "Inequality and Mortality" *International Journal of Health Services* (1983): 102.

During the colonial era the focus was on the health problems of the broad categories outlined in the above paragraphs. Today however, there is growing awareness that within these categories, the health of certain groups is deteriorating faster than that of the generality. Within the rural areas, for example, the plight of women, children, and the elderly is a case in point. Generally it was the woman who remained in the rural areas to farm, take care of the children and the elderly, and do the housework. An increasing number of households are being headed by women.[78] These are the rural households most likely to be in a state of crises. Many do not receive the expected financial support from the migrant spouse; they also cannot count on as much support from the extended family as each household withdraws from the larger unit to fend more for itself. More cash is now needed to purchase many items, but women are less able to secure the more lucrative rural jobs. Data from Botswana reveal that children—especially female children—in households headed by women are more likely to have nutritional problems than in other households.[79] In Nigeria, it has been reported also that the farming duties of a wife which had developed under the precapitalist system have been harnessed to assist the husband in the production of cash crops, while the old forms of compensation have been discarded.[80] Thus a wife though working long hours on the cocoa or tobacco farm no longer has a direct share in the proceeds as she still does with food crop production. In addition, many women lament the fact that the amount of time required on the cash crop farm interferes with their other income-earning activities.

A study conducted by Ekpenyong et al. among elderly (over 60 years) Nigerians in southwestern and eastern Nigeria concluded that although the elderly still receive assistance from family members, rural dwellers are the most likely to be in a crisis situation. Thus "ironically, it may be becoming more difficult to maintain family life in villages with large scale out-migration than in the cities and 'abandoned old people' may be more common in the former than in the latter."[81] Among this group of citizens not only do rural dwellers have more problems than urbanites, but women have more difficulties than men. For instance rural widows are more likely than widowers to be saddled with grandchildren sent from the cities. This responsibility is increasingly found to be difficult. Rural females also report more health complaints than other respondents. They are followed by rural men, urban women, and urban men.

The desperate situation of certain groups within the rural areas was succinctly summarized by Chambers et al. in their findings from a seminar on rural poverty and health in the less developed countries. Included in their survey were Gambia, Nigeria, Tanzania, Kenya, and Mali. It was concluded that climatic factors notwithstanding, the new economic relationships which developed between rich and poor peasant households were important contributions to health problems in the rural areas. One may add also that while the cost of all goods has been rising, those of non-farm goods have risen faster than farm goods. Again, the rural economy does not receive an adequate share of investment considering its role in producing revenue. The situation in these areas is that the weaker groups carry the heaviest burdens. Thus, afflicted by sickness, pregnancies and births, short of food, with food prices high, and with a high need for energy for agricultural work, the poorer people are often driven to distress sales or borrowing. They sell or mortgage land, livestock, jewellery, their future crop, or their labour; they beg from patrons; they become indebted to money lenders. The seasonal crisis drives them to dependency.[82]

Women and their children as well as the elderly were over-represented in this group.

The industrial workers in the cities and mines are another major group causing concern. During the colonial period mines were an established feature of many colonies, but heavy industry was generally discouraged. Now, however, interest in building such concerns is growing rapidly. Since the 1920s medical and social science research in Europe and America has exposed the link between industrial pollution and various diseases. In the industrialized nations, government legislation and consumer group agitations have made it very difficult for manufacturers to operate with the profit margins to which they had become accustomed.[83] The solution for many businesses has been to transfer their enterprise to a less developed nation where fewer regulations exist, the enforcement of them is weak, and government's overriding concern is to attract investment. The asbestos story is the most notorious. Myers has traced the politics of the asbestos business to the present situation in which a substantial portion of the world output of asbestos materials comes from South Africa.[84] While countries like Britain sold their mines to be rid of the mounting problems, others like Western Germany transferred asbestos factories to South Africa. Diseases related to exposure are lung cancer, asbestosis, and mestotheliomia. As expected, better care is taken of the health of industrial white workers than Africans. Other hazardous items include pesticides and outmoded equipment.[85]

Therefore the African industrial worker is exposed to both the types of industrial disorders prevalent among Western workers as well as the communicable and nutritional diseases common in non-Western societies.[86] The double burden being endured is not merely an additive one. Rather the interaction of the two situations devastates the worker. Thus the urban black worker in South Africa while continuously exposed to infectious diseases such as tuberculosis, venereal diseases, and pneumonia now contends with industrial problems such as accidents, silicosis, and lung cancer.[87]

In summarizing the health situation for the post-colonial period one can argue that the situation has remained serious. In the rural areas where from 60 percent to 80 percent of the people live, many households are caught in a downward spiral of growing poverty, deteriorating health, and more poverty. The volume of communicable diseases is high for the lower strata of the various nations. In addition, nutritional problems such as kwashiorkor and marasmus are often on the increase. News bulletins in Nigeria now report the establishment of special malnutrition clinics in some of the government hospitals to handle the unprecedented volume of nutritional disorders among children. Recently in Lagos, the president of the Pediatric Association of Nigeria reported that formerly rare nutritional disorders, such as Canorum Oris, have now become common.[88] In subsaharan Africa, maternal mortality remains high. There are more than ten maternal deaths per 1,000 live births in most countries including the Congo, Ethiopia, the Gambia, Nigeria, Lesotho, and Somalia.[89] In Nigeria it is between ten in the urban centers and twenty-five in the rural areas. The problem of malnutrition for child bearing women complicates a situation already saturated by infectious diseases and overwork. While the elite are able to escape the full impact of diseases of poverty, there is some indication that the disorders of affluence (gout, hypertension, diabetes, and the effects of bleaching preparations) are appearing.[90] Nevertheless, the pattern of disease has not changed much since the precolonial era. This is in contrast to the West where the pattern has changed from infectious to chronic/degenerative diseases.

Summary

Health remains one of the most fundamental values in society. At the group level, it is both an expression of a group's overall ability to command resources as well as a resource itself for securing other values (education, agricultural output, children/ biological reproduction).[91] Disease outbreak is therefore not a random biological phenomenon. The growing anxiety about the health of African populations is due precisely to the belief that the majority are increasingly unable to obtain the necessary resources to make a difference. From the precolonial to the post-colonial period communities have moved from a state of relative self-sufficiency to one in which the terms for survival are manipulated elsewhere (both abroad and by the national elite). Thus the price paid for agricultural goods, the percentage of the budget re-invested in the rural areas, the cost of imported manufactured articles, and the planning of health services work to the disadvantage rural dwellers and the urban poor. When the above are combined with indigenous patriarchal institutions, such as female circumcision and female domestic and farm work, or with the new industrial health hazards, the result is grim.

In this chapter it has been noted that in addition to the growing health inequalities existing among African and Western populations, the trend has also been one of increased health inequalities among segments of African populations. These inequalities can be traced to the complex of economic, political, and familial relationships existing between the interacting segments. Thus morbidity and mortality patterns remain rooted in the problem of poverty, while the volume of each remains high for all but a few privileged groups.

NOTES

1. R. Taussig, "Reification and the Consciousness of the Patient," *Social Science and Medicine* 14B (1980): 3-13; A. Young, "The Anthropologies of Illness and Sickness," *Ann. Rev. Anthropol.* 11 (1982): 257-85.
2. P. Abrams, *Historical Sociology* (Somerset: Open Books, 1982).
3. R. Duff and A. Hollingshead, *Sickness and Society* (New York: Harper and Row, 1968); R. Hurley, "The Health Crisis of the Poor," in *The Social Organization of Health* ed. H. Dreitzel (New York: MacMillan, 1971), pp. 83-122; D. Maier, "Nineteenth Century Asante Medical Practices," *Comparative Studies in Society and History* 21/1 (1979): 3-81.
4. E. Stark, "The Epidemic as a Social Event," *International Journal of Health Services* 7/4 (1977): 681-705.
5. A. Mabogunje and P. Richards, "Land and People: Models of Spatial and Ecological Processes in West African History," in *History of West Africa*, vol. 1, ed. A. Ajayi and M. Crowther (London: Longman, 1971), pp. 5-47.
6. Abrams, *Historical Sociology*; N. Elias, *What is Sociology?* (London: Hutchinson, 1970).
7. S. Clarke, *Marx, Marginalism and Modern Sociology* (London: MacMillan, 1982).
8. O. Woodham-Smith, *The Great Hunger* (London: New English Library, 1962); F. Cartwright, *Disease and History* (London: Rupert Hart-Davis, 1972); Stark, "The Epidemic."
9. H. Zinsser, *Rats, Rice and History* (Boston: Little Brown, 1934).
10. G. Hartwig, *The Art of Survival in East Africa* (New York: Africana Publishing Corporation, 1976); P. Lovejoy, "The Internal Trade of West Africa Before 1800," in *History of West Africa*, vol. 1, ed. A. Ajayi and M. Crowther (London: Longman, 1971), pp. 648-90.

11. P. Curtin, "Epidemiology and the Slave Trade," *Political Science Quarterly* 83/2 (1968): 190-216. Reference on p. 199.
12. J. Macquet, *The Premise of Inequality in Ruanda* (London: Oxford University Press, 1961).
13. T. McKelvey, *Man Against TseTse* (Ithaca: Cornell University Press, 1973), p. 57.
14. Curtin, "Epidemiology."
15. D. Jilek-Aall, "Kifafa: A Tribal Disease in an East African Bantu Population," in *Anthropology and Mental Health* (The Hague: Mouton, 1976), pp. 57-66.
16. J. Goody, *Technological Tradition and the State in Africa* (London: Oxford University Press, 1971).
17. W. Clarence-Smith, "Slaves, Commoners and Landlords in Bulozi, c. 1875 to 1906," *Journal of African History* 20 (1979): 219-34.
18. Macquet, *Premise of Inequality*.
19. H. Tedlie, "Materia Medica and Diseases," in *Mission from Cape Coast to Ashantee (1819)*, by T. Bowdich (London: Frank Cass, 1966), pp. 370-80.
20. Maier, "Nineteenth Century Asante Medical Practices."
21. Sen in L. Tilly, "Food Entitlement, Famine and Conflict," *Journal of Interdisciplinary History* 14/2 (1983): 333-48.
22. P. Talbot, *Peoples of Southern Nigeria*, vol. 3 (London: Frank Cass, 1926.
23. O. Onwubiko, *History of West Africa* (Onitsha: Africana Publishers, 1967).
24. McKelvey, *Man Against TseTse*.
25. G. Hartwig, "Smallpox in the Sudan," *International Journal of Historical Studies* 14/1 (1981): 5-33.
26. Zinsser, *Rats, Rice and History*; Cartwright, *Disease and History*.
27. R. Grosse, "Interrelation Between Health and Population: Observations Derived from Field Experiences," *Social Science and Medicine* 14C/2 (1980): 99-120.
28. G. Howe, *Man, Environment and Disease in Britain* (New York: Barnes and Noble, 1972).
29. T. Zeldin, *France 1848-1945* (Oxford: Clarendon Press, 1977).
30. World Bank, *World Development Report 1984* (New York: Oxford University Press, 1984).

31. N. Ball, "Drought and Dependence in the Sahel," *International Journal of Health Service* 8/2 (1978): 271-98.
32. B. Davidson, *Africa in Modern History* (Harmondsworth: Penguin Books, 1978); T. Aidoo, "Rural Health Under Colonialism and Neo-Colonialism: a Survey of the Ghanian Experience," *International Journal of Health Service* 12/4 (1982): 637-57.
33. R. Shenton, and M. Watts, "Capitalism and Hunger in Northern Nigeria," *Review of African Political Economy* 15-16 (1980): 53-62.
34. J. McCracken, "Experts and Expertise in Colonial Malawi," *African Affairs* 81/322 (1982): 101-116; A. Beck, *A History of the British Medical Administration of East Africa, 1900-1950* (Cambridge: Harvard University Press, 1970); Mabogunje and Richards, "Land and People"; M. Turshen, "The Impact of Colonialism on Health and Health Services in Tanzania," *International Journal of Health Service* 7/1 (1977): 8-35.
35. B. Brown, "Impact of Male Labour Migration on Women in Botswana," *African Affairs* 82/328 (1983): 367-88.
36. G. Arrighi, "Labour Supplies in Historical Perspective: Proletarization of the African Peasantry in Rhodesia," *Journal of Development Studies* 6 (1970): 197-234; S. Feierman, "Struggles for Control: The Social Roots of Health and Healing in Modern Africa," *African Studies Review* 28/2-3 (1985): 73-147; J. Bujra, "Class, Gender and Capitalist Transformation in Africa," *African Development* 8/3 (1983): 17-42.
37. D. Doyal, *The Political Economy of Health* (Boston: South End Press, 1979).
38. Feierman, "Struggles for Control."
39. N. Dixon-Fyle, "Reflections on Economic and Social Change Among the Plateau Tonga of Northern Rhodesia c. 1890-1935," *International Journal of African Historical Studies* 16/3 (1983): 423-39.
40. M. Doornbos, "Ethnicity, Christianity and the Development of Social Stratification in Colonial Ankole, Uganda," *International Journal of African Historical Studies*, 9/4 (1976): 555-75; R. Shenton, *The Development of Capitalism in Northern Nigeria* (Toronto: University of Toronto Press, 1986).

41. Doornbos, "Ethnicity."
42. C. Bakwesegba, "Patterns, Causes and Consequences of Polarized Development in Uganda," in *Urbanization, National Development and Regional Planning in Africa*, ed. S. El-Shakha and B. Obundho (New York: Praeger, 1974), pp. 47-65. Reference on p. 54.
43. E. Abdin et al., *A World of Differentials* (London: Hodder and Stoughton, 1983).
44. R. Stren, "The Evolution of Housing Policy in Kenya," in *Urban Challenge in East Africa* ed J. Hutton (Nairobi: East African Publishing House, 1972), p. 76.
45. L. Vail and D. White, *Capitalism and Colonialism in Mozambique* (London: Heineman, 1980), p. 315.
46. C. Uche, "The Contexts of Mortality in Nigeria," *Genus* 37/1-2 (1981): 123-35.
47. D. Gamble, "Infant Mortality Rates in Rural Areas in The Gambia Protectorate," *Journal of Tropical Medicine and Hygiene* 55 (1952): 145-49.
48. Sierra Leone, *Report of the Census for the Year 1931* (Freetown: Government Printer, 1931).
49. J. Lasker, *Health Care Society in the Ivory Coast: An Approach to the Study of National Health Systems*, Ph.D. diss., Harvard University, Cambridge, Massachusetts, 1976.
50. C. Hughes, and J. Hunter, "Disease and 'Development' in Africa," in *Social Organization of Health* ed. H. Dreitzel (New York: MacMillan, 1971), pp. 151-214.
51. Shenton and Watts, "Capitalism and Hunger."
52. Uche, "Contexts of Mortality,"; B. Nicol, "Fertility and Food in Northern Nigeria," *The West African Medical Journal* 8/1 (1959): 18-27. Data by Calletti et al. are cited in Uche and Nicol.
53. A. Aderibigbe ed., *Lagos: The Development of an African City* (London: Longman, 1975).
54. Federal Ministry of Health Report for 1955.
55. B. Jewziewicki, "The Great Depression and the Making of the Colonial Economic System in the Belgian Congo," *African Economic History* 4 (1977): 153-76; Davidson, *Africa in Modern History*.
56. Vale and White, *Capitalism and Colonialism*.
57. World Bank, *World Development Report 1984*.

58. World Bank, *World Development Report 1984*.
59. L. Cliffe, and R. Moorsom, "Rural Class Formation and Ecological Collapse in Botswana," *Review of African Political Economy* 15-16 (1979): 35-52; Ball, "Drought and Dependence,"; O. Schuftan, "Foreign Aid and Its Role in Maintaining the Exploitation of the Agricultural Sector: Evidence from a Case Study in Africa," *International Journal of Health Service* 13/1 (1983): 33-49; S. Berry, "Oil and the Disappearing Peasantry: Accumulation, Differentiation and Underdevelopment in Western Nigeria," *African Economic History* 13 (1984): 1-22.
60. E. Osagbae, "Food Culture and the Development Process in Nigeria," paper presented at the Seminar of Nigerian Food Culture, University of Ibadan, 1986.
61. S. Amin et al., "The Social Sciences and the Development Crisis in Africa," *African Development* 3/4 (1978): 423-45; H. Alavi, "The Structure of Peripheral Capitalism," in *The Sociology of "Developing Societies"* ed. H. Alavi and T. Shanin (London: MacMillan, 1982); M. Brown, "Developing Societies as Part of an International Political Economy," in *Sociology of "Developing Societies"* ed. H. Alavi and T. Shanin (London: MacMillan, 1982), pp. 153-71; R. Kapinsky, "Capitalist Accumulation in the Periphery: The Kenyan Case," *Review of African Political Economy* 17 (1980): 83-105.
62. S. El-Shakha, "Development Planning in Africa: An Introduction," in *Urbanization, National Development and Regional Planning*, ed. S. El-Shakha and R. Obocho; Lasker, *Health Care*; D. Bello-Iman, "Inequality in Social Infrastructural Provisions in Relation to Health Facilities in Nigeria," paper presented at the National Conference on Inequality and Social Policy held at the University of Ife, Ile-Ife, 1984; Aidoo, "Rural Health Under Colonialism."
63. J. Gugber, and W. Flanagan, *Urbanization and Social Change in West Africa* (Cambridge: Cambridge University Press, 1978), pp. 41-42.
64. Lasker, *Health Care*, p. 138.
65. A. Olokesusi, "Improving the Quality of Life in Rural Nigeria Through Enhanced Health Care Delivery Systems," paper presented at the National Conference on rural Productivity

213

and Quality of Life in a Depressed Economy, University of Ife, Ile-Ife, 1986.

66. H. Hopkins, *Egypt: The Crucible* (London: Sedher and Warburg, 1969).

67. T. Pearce, "Political and Economic Changes in Nigeria and the Organization of Medical Care," *Social Science and Medicine* 14B/2 (1980): 91-98.

68. B. Mburu, "Health Systems as Defenses Against the Consequences of Poverty: Equity in Health as Social Justice," *Social Science and Medicine* 17/16 (1983): 1149-57; B. Okuneye, "Have Agricultural Cooperatives Really Bridged the Gap Between the Rich and the Poor?" paper presented at the National Conference on Inequality and Social Policy, the University of Ife, Ile-Ife, 1984.

69. A. Hake, *African Metropolis* (Brighton: Susex University Press, 1977).

70. Abdin et al., *A World of Differentials* (London: Hodder and Stoughton, 1983).

71. I. Markovitz, *Power and Class in Africa* (Englewood Cliffs: Prentice Hall, 1977).

72. Cliffe and Moorsom, "Rural Class Formation."

73. Okuneye, "Have Agricultural Cooperatives," p. 8.

74. Department of Demography and Social Statistics, *Effects of Modernisation on Family and Demographic Behaviour in Oyo State, Nigeria*, research report submitted to the Rockefeller Foundation, 1986; I. Ekanam, and G. Farooq, "The Dynamics of Population Change in Southern Nigeria," *The Nigerian Journal of Economic and Social Studies* 18/1 (1976): 51-77.

75. J. Gregory and V. Piche, "Inequality and Mortality: Demographic Hypothesis Regarding Advanced and Peripheral Capitalism," *International Journal of Health Services* 13/1 (1983): 89-106.

76. D. Ekanem and J. Ebigbola, "Levels, Patterns and Trends of Mortality in South Western Nigeria," in *National Survey of Fertility and Family Planning*, ed. L. Adeokun (Ile-Ife: Ife University, 1979); T. Pearce and Tarwa Odebiyi, "The Impact of Socio-economic Inequalities on Health: The Double Burden of the Nigerian Poor," *African Development* 4/4 (1979): 64-83.

77. B. Unterhalter, "Inequalities in Health and Disease: The Case of Mortality Rates for the City of Johannesburg, South Africa 1910-1979," *International Journal of Health Services* 12/4 (1982): 617-36; B. Unterhalter, "The Health of the Urban Black in the South African Context," *Social Science and Medicine* 16/11 (1982): 1111-17.

78. Cliffe and Moorsom, "Rural Class Formation"; E. Ivan-Smith, ed., *Link In*, newsletter (London: Commonwealth Secretariat, 1986).

79. Brown, "Impact of Male Labour Migration."

80. O. Aina, *Relative Time Allocation Between Women's Multiple Roles: A Case Study of Yoruba Peasant Women in Cocoa Production*, Ph.D. diss., Department of Sociology/ Anthropology, University of Ife, Ile-Ife, 1985.

81. O. Ekpenyong et al., "Nigerian Elderly: A Rural-Urban and Interstate Comparison," *African Frontology* 5 (1987): 5-17. Reference on p. 17.

82. R. Chambers, et al., "Seasonal Dimensions to Rural Poverty: Analysis and Practical Implications," *Journal of Tropical Medicine and Hygiene* 82/8 (1979): 156-72. Reference in on p. 159.

83. R. Elling, "Industrialization and Occupational Health in Underdeveloped Countries," *International Journal of Health Services* 7/2 (1977): 209-235.

84. J. Myers, "The Social Context of Occupational Disease: Asbestos and South Africa," *International Journal of Health Services* 11/2 (1981): 227-45.

85. R. Elling, "The Capitalist World-System and International Health," *International Journal of Health Services* 11/1 (1981): 21-51.

86. Elling, "Industrialization."

87. H. Seftel, "Diseases in Urban and Rural Black Populations," *South Africa Medical Journal* 51/5 (1977): 121-23; Unterhalter, "Health of the Urban Black."

88. "Health Report," *Daily Times* 19 February 1987, pp. 9, 13.

89. F. Sai, "Family Planning and Maternal Health Care: A Common Goal," *World Health Forum* 7/4 (1986): 315-24.

90. O. Olusi, "The Health of the Ancients," paper presented at the Institute of Cultural Studies, University of Ife, Ile-Ife, 1987.

91. T. Pearce, "Equality in Access to Medical Care: A Review of Nigeria's Approach to Health Preaction," *Ife Social Sciences Review* 7/1-2 (1984): 156-66.

11

NATIONAL GOVERNMENTS AND HEALTH SERVICE POLICY IN AFRICA

Robert Stock and Charles Anyinam

Introduction

Although health conditions in Africa have improved over the past few decades, they remain among the worst in the world. Infective and parasitic diseases account for the bulk of the mortality and morbidity. The disease problems of children, with malnutrition interacting with intestinal helminths, gastroenteritis, and other communicable diseases are particularly severe. Infant mortality is high, not only in low-income economies (129 per 1,000 live births in 1984) but also in countries with lower middle income levels (107 per 1,000 live births).[1]

Many of the determinants of health are also in a poor state. Service coverage of water supply and sanitation, for example, remains poor in many parts of Africa, especially in the rural areas. The percentage of the population with access to safe water ranges from 6 percent in Ethiopia to 46 percent in the Sudan.[2] Although the per capita availability of physicians and other medical personnel has improved substantially in most countries since independence, many still have exceptionally high population to physician ratios (for example 88,000:1 in Ethiopia and 53,000:1 in Malawi in 1983).[3] Much remains to be accomplished.

Each of the more than fifty African states has devised a unique combination of policies designed to improve the health of its population. Health policies have varied significantly in terms of the percentage of budgetary resources allocated to health, the mix of private and public sector health care, the relative emphasis given to curative and preventative medicine, the types of health facilities

217

constructed, the kinds of health workers trained, and the degree of integration of health with related developmental sectors. Moreover, health policies have changed over time in response to the changing nature of the state and the growth of our collective knowledge about potential models for improving health care and health. Three basic health policy models may be identified: a colonial model, a basic health services model, and a primary health care model. These approaches have emerged sequentially, but have tended to be implemented as add-ons to the existing system. Thus, health systems in Africa are "hybrid" rather than "pure model" systems.

A variety of influences affect the shape of health policies and the ability of the state to effectively implement its vision for development. Health policies strongly reflect the priorities and the self-interest of the ruling classes and are significantly influenced by a self-interested medical establishment. Among other things, the successful implementation of policy depends on the administrative capacity of the state. The quantity and types of available resources which can be mobilized significantly affects the range of choices for health policy and the ability to implement them. The sociocultural environment, the nature of the existing health care system, and external influences also have an impact on health policy choices.

This chapter focuses on political influences as they affect the development and implementation of health policies. It is clearly impossible to analyze all the approaches used in every country. Rather, our aim is to search for some generalizations which will permit the classification and comparison of policies used in African states. Conclusions are drawn from the relative mix of different health policy models, the underlying philosophy of the state on health in development, and the relationship between theory and practice.

The development of health policy is examined in three types of states, namely African capitalist, populist socialist, and Afro-Marxist. This three-fold classification is derived from Crawford Young's book *Ideology and Development in Africa*,[4] and resembles other scholars' classifications of African political systems.[5] Although the correlation between political ideology and health policies is far from perfect, it is clear that particular types of states tend to adopt particular approaches to health policy. The other factors listed above—resources, the sociocultural environment, prevailing health care models, and external influences—are often useful in explaining gaps between theory and practice. The chapter moves from a discussion of three types of health policy models to a brief consideration of determinants of health policy in Africa and ends with a comparison of health policies in capitalist, populist socialist, and Afro-Marxist states.

Health Policy Models

Policies on the health of African states stem from three basic models: colonial, basic health services, and primary health care. Elements of each have been adopted in virtually every country without any significant attempt to restructure the health care system. The introduction of a new model has meant the addition of a new level of health care with the existing system remaining otherwise virtually intact.

This study makes occasional reference to indigenous medical systems which predated the colonial conquest and which continue to provide the bulk of health care for most Africans. Our brief consideration of traditional medicine reflects the scanty development of government policy about traditional medicine. Recently, there has been greater interest in ways of fostering the development of traditional medicine as a recognized integral part of the health care system.[6]

The Colonial Model. The colonial state had three priorities, namely, the maintenance of social control, the extraction of sufficient funds to cover administrative costs and ideally generate a surplus, and support for European businessmen engaged in trade and production. Colonial expenditure on health care, although severely constrained due to policies emphasizing self-sufficiency, contributed significantly to these objectives.[7]

The first objective of colonial health care policy was to protect European health, Africa having become "the white man's grave." Hospitals were constructed in the major cities to provide health care first for European officials and later for non-official Europeans. Public health measures undertaken in urban areas, including the maintenance of an unsettled *cordon sanitaire* between European and non-European quarters, drainage improvements and vegetation clearance to reduce insect populations, and

219

numerous edicts to regulate the movement and economic activities of Africans, protected Europeans from the perceived health threat of the African masses. Public health measures also served as means of social control; Africans were subject to intimidation and fines for alleged violations of these regulations.[8]

Colonial health services also provided some rudimentary health care for Africans employed by the colonial state, in European companies, and by individual Europeans. Some basic health services, both curative and preventative, were also provided in areas of economic development such as mining enclaves and export crop regions to ensure greater levels of labor productivity.[9] However, there were also numerous examples, particularly in the early colonial period and from Portuguese, French, and Belgian colonies, of "development" policies which completely ignored the health of African workers and treated them as a literally disposable factor of production.[10] Colonial medicine also gave priority to campaigns against certain diseases such as sleeping sickness, yaws, and malaria. These disease-specific campaigns helped to enhance economic productivity and increase social control. Their apparent benefits for Africans must be weighed against the role of colonial policies which fostered epidemic outbreaks of diseases such as sleeping sickness and syphilis.[11]

Colonial health policy gave scant regard to the health needs of rural Africans in areas with low levels of export crop production. The scattered rural health care facilities were established by local government authorities and financed by tax levies or by missionaries who combined medical care and Christian prosetalization.[12] At the end of the colonial era, most rural Africans had no effective access to Western health care. They continued to rely on traditional medicine which the colonial state either ignored or outlawed, in part because spiritual healers and healing cults could become foci for political protest. In summary, the colonial health system was fragmented in its structure, urban-biased, primarily curative rather preventative and dedicated to serving the diverse needs of the European colonial rulers. The somewhat accelerated growth of health-related expenditure during the last few years of colonial rule brought no fundamental change to this entrenched model.

Following independence, African governments moved to increase the availability of health services primarily adhering to

220

colonial practice. Because few indigenous physicians had been trained during the colonial era, there was a continuing reliance on expatriate doctors. Hence, the training of indigenous medical personnel assumed a high priority. National teaching hospitals were established in most counties for this purpose. Often established as foreign aid projects, these facilities were designed to reproduce the technical medicine of the industrialized countries, rather than to address as a primary concern the most urgent indigenous health problems. These "disease palace" teaching hospitals served to perpetuate the curative, urban, and hierarchical characteristics of colonial health care systems. They also severely distorted national budgets: J.F. Kennedy Hospital in Monrovia, for example, takes some 45 percent of Liberia's expenditure on health care.[13]

The Basic Health Services Model. After independence, many countries sought to expand health care services in both rural and urban areas by constructing additional clinics and hospitals. However, the scarcity of financial and personnel resources limited the ability of national governments to respond to widespread agitation for improved health care. One response to these constraints was the development of a basic health services model.[14] Much of the development and refinement of this approach occurred in Kenya during the 1960s.[15] Later, it was widely adopted in other parts of Africa.

The basic health services model focused primarily on rural health care and gave increased emphasis to preventative medicine, to the role of paraprofessional health care workers, and to the integration of the health care service hierarchy. The basic service unit was the rural health center, commonly staffed by a team of paraprofessionals and without a physician. The delivery of curative and preventative medicine was to be integrated; preventative programs such as health education and maternal and child care were emphasized. With the catchment area of each rural health center, several health clinics would be established to deliver basic health care needs to local populations and to facilitate the referral of more seriously ill patients to a rural health center. Mobile clinics would take health care to the people in more remote locations.[16] This hierarchy of rural health facilities was designed to replace the simple bush dispensaries of colonial health care systems. The higher echelons of health care hierarchy, the regional and national hospitals where difficult cases could be referred for specialist treatment, remained essentially untouched.

Several organizing principles were applied in the design of basic health services systems. Since health care utilization rates decreased at an exponential rate with increasing distance from a facility, health care had to be spatially accessible.[17] Populations located more than approximately eight kilometers from a facility could be served with mobile clinics. A second need was to achieve an optimum size and output for rural health centers. The Kenyan experience suggested that the catchment area for each health center should contain about 20,000 people who would make an average of 2.5 consultations per year.[18] With an optimum spacing of health centers, fewer hospitals would be needed, and these hospitals then could concentrate on specialist and inpatient care. The benefits of careful planning would be greater efficiency in the use of scarce health-system resources and reduced travelling costs for patients.

The basic health services model represented a significant change in favor of rural health needs and health education. Nevertheless, it remained very much a delivery oriented model which focused on the role of professional and paraprofessional health personnel. There was no explicit role for traditional practitioners. Moreover, it did not explicitly address broader issues related to health development, such as the provision of safe water and the improvement of agricultural productivity.

Primary Health Care: Health by the People. The basic health services model introduced important ideas about restructuring priorities in national health care systems to emphasize greater equity and effectiveness. Nevertheless, various problems persisted including the scarcity and maldistribution of resources and the planning of health systems. A joint UNICEF/WHO study published in 1976 identified a long list of obstacles to effective health care provision.[19] These obstacles included inadequate and maldistributed resources for health, inadequate health education, lack of basic sanitation and safe water supplies, lack of clear national health policies, failure to plan for the entire health system as a single entity, opposition from professional bodies to health policy

222

changes, inappropriate training of health personnel, and inadequate community involvement in health care.

These issues were addressed in the UNICEF/WHO conference on primary health care at Alma-Ata in the Soviet Union in 1978. The Alma-Ata Declaration, which defined the meaning of primary health care and urged its adoption as a means to achieve "health care for all by the year 2000," has been recognized as one of the most important statements of principle for the organization of Third World health care.[20] Primary health care was to reflect the economic, sociocultural, and political characteristics of a community. Promotive, preventative, and rehabilitative care were to be emphasized, with priority being given to those in greater need. Health sector planning was to be integrated into the broader scheme of community and regional development along with agriculture, education, housing, water provision and other socio-economic sectors. Primary health care also stressed community and individual self reliance and the full utilization of available resources. Community health services were to be delivered by health care workers locally selected and appropriately trained, ideally including traditional healers. This did not imply the creation of a separate health care system. It recognized the important supportive role of health care professional working in higher order health facilities.

The primary health care model was revolutionary in concept. It redefined health and health policy; instead of viewing them as discrete entities, it incorporated everything impacting on individual and community well-being. It also emphasized local solutions using local resources, and therefore deemphasized the role of medical professionals in local health care. It acknowledged the importance of traditional practitioners. The stress on local control and decision-making challenged the predominant top-down mechanisms of control, and pointed toward the development of a more egalitarian society.[21]

Primary health care was not a new idea. Rather, it grew from the barefoot doctor model which had been so successful in China, and was subsequently introduced into Tanzania, Mozambique, and various other countries.[22] It also reflected the growing preference for integrated development strategies which stressed the potential benefits of bottom-up, rural-based development in place of the dominant trickle-down approaches.[23] The primary health care model often was adopted for reasons other than a commitment to social justice. The emphasis on self-reliance—local communities were to pay the primary health care worker as well as part of the cost of drugs—falsely suggested that primary health care would be economical for the state, permitting an expansion of rural health care without taking resources from the conventional health care system.[24]

Determinants of Health Policy

Health care systems may be organized according to different principles and take various forms. Roemer identifies five types of health systems, namely free enterprise, welfare state, under-developed country, transitional, and socialist.[25] Examples of the last three of these types can be found in Africa.

Studies of health care systems and their determinants have focused on a number of crucial factors. Roemer identified levels of development and socio-political organization as primary determinants; previously he had recognized also the importance of historical and cultural influences.[26] Eyles identified the level of economic development (what may be distributed), the allocation mechanism (how it is distributed), and political identity (why it is distributed in a certain way) as the most important determinants of the shape of health care systems.[27] Allocation mechanisms which may be used to distribute health care resources include the free market, bureaucratic intervention to achieve more equitable distribution in capitalist societies, and central planning.

Although the factors which differentiate health care systems at a global level provide useful guidelines for the analysis of African systems, such factors do not focus on the distinctive nature of African systems. In this study, African health care polices are considered in relation to the nature of the contemporary African states, resource scarcity, sociocultural environments, the existing health care system, and external influences.

The Contemporary African State. Faced with immense demands for improved social services and with the weakness of the capitalist sector African states have had no option but to take the lead in the provision of health care. The state has assumed this dominant role irrespective of whether it has been capitalist, populist socialist, or Afro-Marxist in ideology. The formerly significant mission sector has declined in importance and in many countries has been absorbed into the state sector. The private health care sector has remained small and urban based, although it has recently been growing quickly in wealthier countries such as Nigeria and Kenya.

Despite the pervasiveness of its involvement in economic and social affairs, African states have often been characterized as being weak and ineffective. Many of them suffer from what Callaghy has termed "muddled ideologies," namely poorly-articulated and often contradictory views of how social and economic change should take place.[28] Beyond the articulation of a plan for change lies the challenges of implementation. A "rhetoric-implementation gap" may occur because of the weakness of administrative structures, and dependence on inadequately qualified personnel.[29] Moreover, few regimes rule by popular mandate and some must rely on repressive measures to stay in power. Most states lack both the organizational capacity and popularity needed for sustained and effective popular mobilization, for example, for community development initiatives. Nevertheless, the theory and practice of development in Africa inevitably reflects the overwhelming role of the state and the corresponding weakness of the private sector.

Empirically the state is composed of the executive, legislative, and judicial levels of government, as well as regulatory bodies, parastatals, and other institutions, all of which enforce national sovereignty and carry out public policy. The ideological orientation of the state influences the matrix of socioeconomic policies which it adopts. Within any particular ideological orientation, however, a very wide margin of difference arises from the skill, competence, and rationality with which a given strategy is pursued. The ideological framework is significantly shaped by the dominant classes reflecting their self interest.[30]

In African societies, class dynamics primarily reflect power relations rather than the control of wealth and productive enterprise.[31] The dominant class is the state bourgeoisie, which depends on the state and proximity to political power for survival.[32] The state bourgeoisie is a very powerful conservative force opposing any meaningful redistribution of scarce resources from urban to rural areas or from the rich to the poor.

225

The shape of the contemporary African state significantly reflects the historical legacy of colonial policies and the complex pattern of intersecting class and cultural affiliations. Colonial rule took different forms throughout Africa, leading to economic disparities between colonies and between regions within particular colonies. Colonialism created new political structures and fostered the emergence of new forms of social stratification. New derivative classes composed of clerks, soldiers, teachers, traders, and others whose status and wealth came from participation in the colonial state provided crucial skilled labor and were seen as role models demonstrating the potential rewards of colonial rule. The post-colonial rulers were drawn primarily from these "assimilated" classes.

While colonial underdevelopment and culturally hetero-geneous societies are characteristics of African nations, their manifestation varies greatly from country to country. The evolution and form of contemporary African countries reflect a multitude of local, historical religious, cultural, and geographical circumstances, as well as external links. Therefore, while generalizations may be made about their characteristics in relation to the organization of production and dominant classes, strictly economic determinist explanations, which ignore the distinct histories of particular African states and fail to recognize the diverse forms development can take, are to be avoided.

Theory and Practice: Further Constraints. The choices of African states concerning health care are constrained in relation to resources. Poverty is more pervasive in Africa than in any other continent, with the possible exception of Libya, no African country is prosperous by international standards. Nevertheless, there are significant differences in wealth between Africa's more prosperous states such as Nigeria and Ivory Coast, a middle group of comparatively poor nations such as Ghana and Senegal, and destitute countries such as Ethiopia and Burkina Faso.

Declining terms of trade for most African commodities and the onerous burden of international debt have meant that the resources available to most governments have declined significantly in real terms. Resources for health have been affected by the policies of the International Monetary Fund (IMF) which have stipulated that governments must severely curtail social service expenditures as a precondition for their support in debt rescheduling. A significant resource for health care development in some countries has come from foreign aid; in Botswana, for example, 88 percent of development expenditures for health came from this source.[33] The decline in resources for health care not only limits the possibility of expanded coverage and new programs. Cutbacks have caused a shrinkage of existing health systems; some health facilities are without drugs and sometimes without staff.

The shortage of medical personnel of all types also constrains the expansion of health care systems. Educational systems have a limited capacity to train additional personnel, especially in smaller African countries with a small range of medical training facilities. The scarcity of financial and human resources are closely linked. In times of constraint, universities are unable to expand training programs and governments are unable to attract graduates into the state health care system. Instead, physicians emigrate or go into private practice to serve the rich.

Sociocultural environments vary between and within particular countries, and may impinge upon the development of effective health care delivery systems. For example, the distribution of population constrains choice, particularly in low-density regions. The delivery of health care to nomadic populations has always posed special problems. African countries vary in terms of cultural homogeneity and harmony. To be effective, health programs need to be designed with sensitivity to the cultural milieu in which they are applied. In culturally diverse societies, care must be taken to adapt health care programs to particular ethnic cultural groups. Regional, ethnic, religious, and political-ideological conflicts have occurred, and continue to occur, in numerous African states. Such conflicts may have a profound impact on health; they disrupt economic activity, divert resources from social development to arms purchases, result in the destruction of health facilities, and force people to flee as refugees.

Any existing health care system exerts an active influence on the further development of the system. The existing system exists both as a set of resources and as a familiar model. In Africa the spatial distribution of health care systems remains highly uneven in terms of both space and social class. However, the possibilities for the significant restructuring of the system are limited because of the immobility of existing health care facilities and health-

227

preserving infrastructure such as water supply systems. Other elements, for example human and financial resources, also are relatively immobile, largely because the ruling classes who benefit from the maldistribution of resources are reluctant to sacrifice in the interest of social justice. The medical establishment is a conservative force which resists any move to reduce its professional dominance.[34] Individual physicians are usually reluctant to serve in rural areas.

The development of African health policies is profoundly affected by external influences as well as internal conditions. In recent years the World Health Organization has taken an active role in promoting innovative health policies, especially primary care. However, the options available to African states are constrained by conditions attached to foreign aid and IMF loan guarantees as well as the weak position of African exports in international commodity markets. Moreover, continuing political and military interference by foreign powers diverts resources from development to armaments, as in Angola, and frustrates the potential emergence of more progressive governments, as in Zaire.

Health Care Policies in African States

African Capitalist States. The majority of African states have adopted a capitalist model of development, either explicitly or implicitly under the rubric of a mixed economy. African capitalist countries like Ivory Coast, Kenya, and Nigeria are characterized by open economics that are centered on the private sector, although state intervention is generally pervasive. The capitalist states have strong relationships with Western industrialized countries. Ivory Coast, for instance, maintains close ties with France and grants privileged status to French nationals and French capital. In terms of economic growth, Ivory Coast and Kenya appear to have a stronger record, even though their economic growth slowed down at the end of the 1970s. African capitalist states permit very high returns to a relatively small segment of the population, in particular businessmen, top functionaries, ruling politicians, and expatriates.

The examples cited in the following discussion are from Nigeria, Kenya, and Senegal, reflecting the greater accessibility of information about these countries' health policies. It should be noted, however, that these countries all have above-average or average levels of development and per capita income. Health policies in these countries have shown a marked continuity from the colonial era to the present. Despite the overall growth of the health sector and expansion of rural health services, there has been no radical change in the structure of their health care systems.

During the 1960s, theories of development and modernization emphasized macro scale economic growth rather than fulfillment of basic needs such as health services. For example, Nigeria's First National Development Plan (1962-1968) allocated only 2.5 percent of federal expenditures to health; actual expenditures on health was only 1.4 percent during the period.[35] Much of the initial expenditure was on teaching hospitals to train physicians to improve access to health care. These facilities were incredibly expensive to construct and maintain, and contributed little to solving the fundamental health problems of the masses. The early emphasis on teaching hospitals reflected the influence of the medical establishment intent on maintaining their professional dominance,[36] aid donors who saw teaching hospitals as a means of promoting future sales of medical technology,[37] and the ruling classes who demanded international standards of health care for themselves and who viewed these hospitals as important symbols of natural progress.[38]

In some countries, rural communities pressured national governments in the years after independence to improve basic services, including health care. These pressures were especially great in countries with electoral political systems. In parts of Nigeria and Kenya, community groups constructed clinics as self-help projects and then sought government help to staff them. The basic health services model was developed in Kenya during the 1960s as a response to popular agitation for better rural health care. This approach was centered on a hierarchical structure of accessible health facilities staffed primarily by paraprofessionals. The basic health services model was later introduced to many other countries of Africa.

Nigeria drafted a particularly ambitious basic health services scheme during its Third National Development Plan (1975-1979).[39] A hierarchical network of twenty health clinics, four primary health centers and one comprehensive health center was to be provided for each 150,000 people. However, progress was slow, even before the dramatic decline in oil prices and the burden of national debt repayment forced severe cutbacks in capital expenditure. In Kano State, for example, only sixty-one of the planned 600 clinics had been constructed as of 1982, and some of these remained closed due to staff shortages.[40] Each unit of twenty clinics and associated health centers had cost eight million Naira, instead of the budgeted 500,000 Naira.[41]

Despite the increase in rural health care provision, the entrenched urban, regional, and class biases were not significantly altered. In Kano State, Nigeria, the doctor-population ratio was 1:286,000 outside the city of Kano, seven years after the launching of the Third National Development Plan.[42] In Senegal, three quarters of the country's physicians and pharmacists serve Dakar, which has only one-fifth of the national population.[43] Dakar's per capita consumption of pharmaceuticals is five times that of rural Senegal. In Kenya, per capita expenditure in 1973-1974 on curative health services was 77.35 Kenyan pounds in Nairobi, but only 3.58 pounds to 14.14 pounds in Kenya's other provinces.[44]

While the basic health services model had stressed the importance of preventative programs, the reality was different. Staff were overburdened by the demand for curative health care. Commitment to prevention as a first priority remained soft at all levels of the system. It was only with the development of the basic needs approach and integrated rural development model during the late 1970s that greater attention was paid to preventative health care. The construction of water supply systems has taken precedence in many countries. More recently WHO's Expanded Programme for Immunization against the common childhood diseases has brought the first sustained commitment to preventative health care in most of rural Africa. Although the primary health care model has been introduced in many capitalist African states during the past decade, development has seldom proceeded beyond the pilot project phase. There are no African capitalist states where this approach has had any real national impact. These failures reflect a lack of serious commitment to rural mobilization and rural transformation.

With the 1980s financial crises of increasing debt and stagnant revenues which have afflicted all of Africa, health care expenditures have been slashed. Several countries have introduced hospital user fees to generate revenue; such fees have created a significant barrier to health care for all but the rich.[45] Austerity has led to the slashing of national drug purchases. The scarcity of drugs has virtually paralyzed the health care system in many rural areas and added to the cost of care for urban patients who purchased prescribed drugs.

The impact of government cutbacks has been much less drastic for those willing and able to pay for the high cost of care. Nigerian hospitals have expanded amenity ward facilities for the rich, and at the same time have slashed budgets for basic health care.[46] Private medical practice continues to expand rapidly in the major cities. Meanwhile, Nigerians spent an estimated U.S. $2.3 million during 1974-1983 to obtain medical treatment abroad.[47] The Nigerian bourgeoisie continue to call for the establishment of a national health insurance scheme.[48] Health policies in African capitalist states strongly reflect the self-interest of the urban-based ruling classes who have no interest in dismantling the inequitable health care systems from which they benefit. As for rural areas, they have been served last and least, and have suffered the greatest cutbacks in health services since the imposition of austerity measures.

Populist Socialist States. Populist socialist regimes are those which espouse socialist principles, but which either do not stress or explicitly reject Marxism.[49] The doctrines of African socialism, as espoused by Nyerere in Tanzania, or by Kaunda in Zambia, were typical of the populist socialist pathway. Ghana under Nkrumah and Guinea under Toure provided the earliest models. These states tended to be nationalist, populist, and anti-capitalist. Development policies stressed the role of state enterprises and concentrated on rural reforms designed to achieve mass mobilization. However, despite the use of radical rhetoric, the populist socialist states are non-Marxist, both in terms of self-identification and development policies.

The populist socialist states have a mixed socioeconomic development record. The Tanzanian economy, for instance, enjoyed some reasonable success during the first decade of independence but was badly hit by excesses of the mass village campaign of the 1970s as well as by drought and by deteriorating terms of trade. Ghana under Nkrumah during the years 1981-1988 had a mediocre economic performance because state-run industrial projects intended as the driving force for development proved unsuccessful and socialist-inspired rural policies were unpopular.

Health services remained extremely poor at the time of independence, especially away from areas of economic development. In Zambia for example, health services were highly concentrated in the copper belt where mining companies had established health facilities for their workers, and in the restricted areas of substantial European settlement.[50] There were also great disparities in Ghana and Tanzania between the health services in urban areas and other pockets of modern development and in the underdeveloped rural peripheries.[51]

The post-independence governments of Tanzania, Zambia, and Ghana had similar visions which included rapid social and economic development and improved quality of life for rural populations. Charismatic leaders—Nkrumah in Ghana, Nyerere in Tanzania, and Kaunda in Zambia—played a crucial role in setting forth national agendas and mobilizing all segments of society to participate in the nation-building process. Their ideologies have been criticized as utopian, vague, and sometimes contradictory, but the far-reaching importance of their visions of independent African development cannot be denied.[52]

Improved health care was an important element in their programs. Following independence, many new hospitals, health centers, and dispensaries were constructed, and many additional medical personnel of all types were trained. In Zambia, for example, the numbers of government hospitals and rural health centers doubled in the first decade after independence.[53] The health care system of Tanzania expanded even more rapidly, from a total of 1,754 health facilities in 1972 to 2,892 in 1976.[54] This expansion occurred primarily in the least-serviced regions, reflecting the emphasis given to equity in development in the Arusha Declaration (1967) and the Second Five Year Plan (1969-1974).

Some aspects of their health policies were quite innovative. Nkrumah attempted to revive indigenous medicine by establishing a research institute to study herbal cures and supporting the establishment of a national association of healers.[55] This official recognition of traditional medicine was a significant departure from colonial policy and occurred some fifteen years before international organizations such as WHO began to acknowledge the importance of traditional practitioners. Tanzania and Zambia have both carried forward Nkrumah's mission with programs to remove colonial legal barriers restricting traditional medicine, promote the study of herbal remedies, and incorporate healers and traditional birth attendants into primary health care.[56] The open-mind attitude toward traditional medicine in Nkrumah's Ghana and in Tanzania and Zambia reflected their ideological emphasis on self-reliance, nationalism, and the affirmation of African identity.

Tanzania had moved to implement key elements of the primary health care approach years before its endorsement in the Alma-Ata Declaration. The development of a primary health care strategy was one consequence of the Arusha Declaration which set forth an agenda for cooperative, self-reliant, egalitarian, and rural-based development for Tanzania.[57] Scattered rural populations were resettled in villages where services such as health care could be provided more efficiently, and where rural people could be encouraged to actively participate in the development process. A program for training primary health care workers, modelled on the Chinese barefoot doctors, was established.[58] National health education programs such as *mtu ni afya* (man in health) and *chakula ni uhai* (food is life) used media presentations and community discussion groups to improve awareness of health and stimulate self-reliant health projects such as latrine construction and mosquito control.[59] Successive studies demonstrated that these programs had increased public awareness of health and modified personal behavior. The relative success of primary health care in Tanzania compared to most countries may be attributed to the favorable political environment, namely the state's commitment to this approach, its implementation as part of a coherent policy of social and economic transformation, and its concern for popular involvement in development.[60] The introduction of primary health care in Zambia, where the state has been much less resolutely committed to rural progress and popular leadership, has been less successful.[61]

Despite a stated commitment in all three countries to a redistribution of health care resources from urban curative medicine to rural health, urban areas continue to receive most expenditures. Tanzania managed to reduce the proportion of the health budget for urban hospitals from 74 percent to 60 percent, and to increase funds for rural health care from 12 percent to 18.5

233

percent between 1970 and 1980.[62] Nevertheless, this shift fell far short of the stated objective of radically redistributing resources in favor of rural needs. Apart from the reluctance of urban elites, including the medical establishment, to reallocate their own privileges, Tanzania also has been constrained in its planning by the large foreign aid component (80 percent of 1982-1983 budgeted expenditure) in the health sector and by the considerable influence which foreign donors exert over the allocation of these funds.[63]

Contemporary trends in the populist socialist countries graphically illustrate the nature and depth of economic problems faced by most African states, and their impacts on social policy and the quality of life. Terms of trade have moved steadily against African countries and frustrated their attempts to manage existing levels of debt. With the collapse of copper prices and the concurrent oil crisis, Zambia's debt service rose from 8 percent of foreign exchange earnings in 1974 to 52 percent in 1983.[64] Zambia, like Tanzania and Ghana, has had to succumb with great reluctance to the IMF's "bitter pill" conditions.

While nominal expenditures on health in Zambia increased from Kwacha 27.2 million in 1970 to Kwacha 73.2 in 1984, there was a massive decline in real expenditure on health, when inflation and evaluation are considered, from Kwacha 21.9 million (16.1 million recurrent and 5.8 million capital) in 1970 to Kwacha 11.9 million (11.6 million recurrent and 0.3 million capital) in 1984.[65] Expansion of the health care system became virtually impossible, and recurrent expenditures for drug supplies, equipment, and salaries were jeopardized. Doctors emigrated *en masse*; their numbers fell from 821 in 1981 to 520 in 1985.[66] Increasingly stringent IMF conditions imposed since 1984 forced even greater reductions in social service expenditures, increasing the cost of basic needs.

Tanzania and Ghana experienced similar economic crises and had to drastically reorient their policies. Ghana introduced user fees for health services, and moved to privatize the distribution of medicines.[67] While the IMF was enthusiastic about the impacts of its bitter pills, these measures brought real suffering, increased health risks, and much reduced access to health care for the poor.[68]

234

The populist socialist states demonstrated a real commitment to improved health care. Health indicators demonstrate the benefits of innovative health policies. However, these gains are threatened by various factors including world commodity markets and international intervention in the planning process. Nkrumah's warnings about neocolonial limitations to African independence proved to be all too accurate.[69]

Afro-Marxist States. Afro-Marxist states are those which maintain an explicit commitment to Marxism-Leninism as the state ideology.[70] Several such states—Mozambique, Angola, Guinea-Bissau, and Zimbabwe—were forged through a process of armed struggle against colonial regimes, guided by a revolutionary vanguard. Other Afro-Marxist regimes, including those of Congo People's Republic, Benin, Burkina Faso, Madagascar, and Ethiopia are more complex. While all are explicitly Marxist-Leninist in ideology, they emerged as a result of military coups rather than prolonged revolutionary struggle. The adoption of Marxist-Leninist principles reflect a variety of influences, including the legacy of ideas from pre-independence socialist parties, the Rassemblement Democratique African (RDA), the disaffection of lower-ranking soldiers of humble origin with the capitalist status quo, and regional and ethnic rivalries particular to each country. The dominant social group in the Afro-Marxist states has been called the "revolutionary democrats" (political figures, intellectuals, and teachers) who are said to be neither tied to capitalism nor allied with multinational capital.

Under this ideological paradigm, there is a consistent thrust to gain control of the "commanding heights" of the economy through state direction. Although these states make efforts to attract Western capital, they generally have extensive ties with communist states. Some of them have performed better economically than their predecessors, but, generally rapid economic growth has eluded them.

Long before their final victories in the anti-colonial armed struggle, the revolutionary Afro-Marxist movements had created distinctive and innovative health care systems. The African Independence Party of Guiné and Cape Verde (PAIGC) maintained a health care system in Guinea-Bissau which was as large as that of the colonial regime. In 1971, they operated a health care system in the liberated areas with over 500 health workers including 70 doctors and with 117 sanitation posts and 9 hospitals.[71] Primary health care workers, trained to deliver basic health care at the community level, formed the backbone of the system. Mobile health brigades provided further support. Preventative medicine and health education received particular emphasis. The PAIGC constitution identified health as a key dimension of socially just development and designated it as a specific responsibility at all levels of the political and administrative structure.[72]

In the liberated areas of Mozambique, the Mozambique Front of Liberation (FRELIMO) maintained an equally developed health care system. Cabo Delgado province, for example, had over 300 FRELIMO health workers in 1972, three years before victory.[73] The system was built upon the village health worker model; primary health care had been practiced for a decade in Mozambique when this model was endorsed by WHO at Alma-Ata. At independence, the challenge of merging two thoroughly different health care systems had to be addressed.[74] The Portuguese colonial officials had virtually ignored health care, except for the white minority concentrated in urban areas. At independence, there were only six prenatal clinics in Portuguese Mozambique. More than two-thirds of the doctors worked in Lorenco Marques. Colonial health care systems were hierarchical, fragmented (emphasizing disease-specific interventions), urban, and curative. In contrast, the liberation forces had developed an integrated approach stressing prevention, focused their attention on rural areas, and built their system around village health workers.

With the collapse of the colonial regime and the nationalization of the health system after independence, five-sixths of the 550 physicians who had worked in colonial Mozambique left.[75] A similar exodus occurred in Angola and Guinea-Bissau. Doctors from Cuba, the Soviet Union, and other socialist countries were employed on an interim basis. The emphasis on primary health care continued since independence. Mozambique trained some 4,500 paramedical workers between 1975 and 1982, enabling it to provide a spatial coverage of health care comparable to that of Kenya and other countries which had been independent for some time.[76]

The new health care systems of Guinea-Bissau, Angola, and Mozambique were developed specifically in relation to ideas of class struggle. In Guinea-Bissau, urban-based bureaucrats were blamed for giving insufficient priority to rural development and spending half of the national health budget in the capital city.[77] Doctors in Mozambique have been reluctant to work in rural areas, and to fully cooperate in the democratization of hospitals.[78] While those committed to egalitarian development have been disturbed by the continuing urban bias in resource allocation, many physicians claim that resources cannot be reallocated to the countryside if urban hospitals are to function. The improvement of the health services of Mozambique and Angola was hampered severely by insurgence fomented by South African, as well as by widespread drought and financial crises. In Mozambique, a large proportion of primary health care workers abandoned their posts, sometimes because their communities were too poor to pay them and sometimes because of the dangers posed by the liberation war.[79]

Mozambique has also assumed an innovative role in the development of basic drug lists to reduce the cost of imported pharmaceuticals. They had published a list of 350 basic drugs to replace the 13,000 varieties formerly imported, and established a system of competitive bidding for drug supply contracts, prior to WHO's endorsement of basic drug schemes.[80] Gish has referred to the gap in Mozambique "between a relatively highly-developed socialist theory and a less well-developed practice."[81] Mozambique and Guinea-Bissau have treated health as a basic human right and a first-order priority. Their commitment has been more than rhetorical; they rank as the top two countries of Africa in terms of the percentage of government expenditures on health.[82]

The development of health policies in Zimbabwe resembles the approach used in the former Portuguese territories. The health care system in pre-independence time was more advanced in terms of numbers of doctors and facilities. However, the typical colonial model prevailed; while white settlers had access to excellent care, blacks particularly in rural areas had only rudimentary health services. Doctor to population ratios of one per 800 whites, compared to one per 62,000 rural Africans were mirrored in infant mortality levels among rural Africans rates which were more than ten times that for urban whites.[83]

At independence, two visions of the future health care system were enunciated.[84] The medical establishment and white settlers emphasized the maintenance of quality care in urban hospitals, the entrenchment of rights for private hospitals and private practice, and counselled against large investment in rural health care. The Zimbabwean government had very different priorities. Their emphasis was on rural health care; 300 rural health centers were planned, and training programs for village health workers established. User fees were eliminated for the poorest 90 percent of the population and restrictions were placed on the expansion of the for-profit medical sector.

The Zimbabwean approach was much less radical in its scope and pace of change than those of Mozambique and Guinea-Bissau. This gradualist approach to health reform has reflected the government's concern with restoring national harmony and economic stability after the long struggle for independence. It seems likely that Zimbabwe will follow a Tanzanian reformist approach stressing rural health care without drastic changes to the urban system, rather than the Mozambican approach of attempting a fundamental restructuring of the health care system.

While the approaches used by the revolutionary Afro-Marxist states show considerable similarity not all of them have demonstrated such dedication to social justice in health. In the Afro-Marxist states which did not emerge through armed struggle, such as Benin and Congo, health has not been singled out as a special priority, and conventional, urban hospital-biased models of health care delivery predominate.[85]

Conclusion

The policy performance of African states, particularly those which appear to determine how and why African states perform as they do, has been the focus of considerable research in recent years. This study has considered the extent to which the health service policies of some African states were influenced by their ideological orientations. While a great range of policy initiatives was adopted in the more than fifty African states, these policies essentially were of three types, namely the colonial, basic health services, and primary health care models. Virtually all states in Africa have health systems incorporating elements of the three modes. The main differences concern the relative mixes of elements of the three models, levels of commitment to social justice in health and in development as a whole, and the willingness to attempt a fundamental restructuring of the health care system. The proportion of budgets allocated to health, the relative expenditures on curative versus preventive medicine, and on urban versus rural health care provide some indication of commitment to the reform of health care systems.

While all African states claim that the health of their citizens is an important priority, there are significant differences in performance. African capitalist states have tended to allocate comparatively small proportions of their budgets to health, and to spend most of their health allocation on urban, curative medicine. The pronounced class biases in access to health care are accentuated by the rapid growth in private sector health care. Populist socialist states have given priority to rural health care and have shown more openness toward non-technological medicine, particularly the primary health care approach, and traditional medicine, than the capitalist states. While some progress was made toward a reallocation of resources toward rural needs and preventive care, urban curative medicine has continued to absorb a disproportionate share of resources. The revolutionary Afro-Marxist states have attempted to restructure their health systems within the larger context of social and economic transformation. While their achievements have been noteworthy, they have fallen far short of objectives.

Statistical indices do not provide conclusive answers concerning the impact of different policy options on the health of Africans. Unfortunately, it is impossible to isolate the effect of ideology from other factors influencing the development and implementation of health policy—differences in the degree of colonial underdevelopment, economic resources and performance, international debt, foreign aid, wars, drought and so on. Thus, comparisons of the infant mortality rates of Nigeria and Mozambique, for example, do not prove that one or the other set of health policies is more effective.

Since the health of Africans reflects so much more than health policy *per se*, it follows that more efficient management of scarce resources or the adoption of new strategies formulated elsewhere in the world are unlikely by themselves to have dramatic effects.[86] The quest for health and the imperative of fundamental political, social, and economic change are inseparable.

NOTES

1. World Bank, *World Development Report 1986* (New York: Oxford University Press, 1986), p. 232.
2. World Bank, *World Development Report*, p. 152.
3. World Bank, *World Development Report*, p. 234.
4. C. Young, *Ideology and Development in Africa* (New Haven: Yale University Press, 1982).
5. J. S. Saul, "Ideology in Africa: Decomposition and Recomposition," in *African Independence: The First Twenty-five Years*, ed. G. M. Carter and P. O'Meara (Bloomington: Indiana University Press, 1985), pp. 300-29.
6. See, for example, C. Good et al., "The Interface of Dual Systems of Health Care in the Developing World: Toward Policy Initiatives in Africa," *Social Science and Medicine* 13D (1979): 141-54.
7. L. Doyal, *The Political Economy of Health* (London: Pluto, 1979).
8. M. Swanson, "The Sanitation Syndrome: Bubonic Plague and Urban Native Health Policy in the Cape Colony, 1900-1909," *Journal of African History* 18 (1977): 387-410.
9. Doyal, *Political Economy*. Also W. Freund, *Capital and Labour in the Nigerian Tin Mines* (Ibadan: Humanities Press, 1981).
10. For a compelling description of the human costs of a colonial development project, see M. A. Azevedo, "The Human Price of Development: The Brazzaville Railway and the Sara of Chad," *African Studies Review* 24 (1981): 1-19.
11. C. C. Hughes and J. M. Hunter, "Disease and 'Development' in Tropical Africa," *Social Science and Medicine* 3 (1970): 443-93, and R. Stock, "Disease and Development on the Underdevelopment of Health: A Critical Review of Geographical Perspectives on African Health Problems," *Social Science and Medicine* 23 (1986): 689-700.

12. T. O. Ranger, "Godly Medicine: The Ambiguities of Medical Missions in Southeast Tanzania," *Social Science and Medicine* 15B (1981): 261-77.
13. H. Nelson (ed.), *Liberia: a Country Study* (Washington: American University, 1981), p. 136.
14. Although "basic health services" and "primary health care" were once used interchangeably, they have had distinctive meanings since the Declaration of Alma-Ata in 1978.
15. N. R. E. Fendall, "Primary Health Care in Developing Countries," *International Journal of Health Services* 2 (1972): 297-315. Also M. King (ed.), *Medical Care in Developing Countries* (New York: Oxford University Press, 1966).
16. R. Jolly and M. King, "The Organization of Health Services," in *Mobile Health Services* by O. Gish and G. Walker (London: Tri-Med, 1977).
17. Jolly and King, "Organization of Health Services." For further detail on the relationship between distance and utilization, see R. Stock, "Distance and the Utilization of Health Services in Rural Nigeria," *Social Science and Medicine* 17 (1983): 563-70.
18. Jolly and King, "Organization of Health Services."
19. V. Djukanovic and E. P. Mach (eds.), *Alternative Approaches to Meeting Basic Health Needs in Developing Countries* (Geneva: World Health Organization, 1975).
20. H. Mahler, "The Meaning of 'Health for All by the Year 2,000,'" *World Health Forum* 2 (1981): 5-22. For a critique of this approach, see O. Gish, "The Political Economy of Primary Health Care and 'Health by the People': an historical exploration," *Social Science and Medicine* 13C (1979): 203-11.
21. R. Start, "Lay workers in primary health care: victims in the process of social transformation," *Social Science and Medicine* 20 (1985): 269-76.
22. V. Sidel and R. Sidel, *Serve the People: Observations on Medicine in the Peoples' Republic of China* (Boston: Beacon Press, 1974).

23. W. B. Stohr and D. R. F. Taylor (eds.), *Development from Above or Below? The Dialectics of Regional Planning in Developing Countries* (New York: Wiley, 1981).

24. Gish, "Political Economy." Also see M. Segall, "Planning and Politics of Resource Allocation for Primary Health Care: Promotion of Meaningful National Policy," *Social Science and Medicine* 17 (1983): 1947-60.

25. M. Il Roemer, *Comparative National Policies on Health Care* (New York: Dekker, 1977).

26. M. I. Roemer, *National Strategies for Health Care Organization* (Ann Arbor: Health Administration Press, 1985).

27. J. Eyles, "Spatial Configurations of Health Care Systems: a Conceptual Approach," paper presented at the third International Symposium in Medical Geography, Kingston, Ontario, 1988.

28. T. M. Callaghy, "The Difficulties of Implementing Socialist Strategies of Development in Africa: The 'First Wave,'" in *Socialism in Sub-Saharan Africa: a New Assessment*, C. G. Rosberg and T. M. Callaghy (Berkeley: Institute of International Studies, University of California, 1979), pp. 112-29.

29. F. M. Mburu, "Rhetoric-Implementation Gap in Health Policy and Health Services Delivery for a Rural Population in a Developing Country," *Social Science and Medicine* 13A (1979): 577-83.

30. C. Young, "Patterns of Social Conflict: State, Class and Ethnicity," *Daedalus* 3/2 (1982): 71-98.

31. R. Sklar, "The nature of class domination in Africa," *Journal of Modern African Studies* 17 (1979): 531-52.

32. Young "Patterns of Social Conflict."

33. B. Hogh and E. Petersen, "The Basic Health and System in Botswana: a Study of the Distribution and Cost in the Period 1973-1979," *Social Science and Medicine* 19 (1984): 783-92.

34. E. Friedson, *Professional Dominance* (New York: Atherton, 1970).

35. F. Abudu, "Planning Priorities and Health Care Delivery in Nigeria," *Social Science and Medicine* 17 (1983): 1995-2002.

36. The dominant attitude of the medical establishment is typified by the advice of Dr. S. L. Adesuyi, Chief Medical

242

Advisor to the Nigerian Government, to a Symposium on Priorities in National Health Planning held in Ibadan in 1973. He strongly advised against training paraprofessionals to take over certain functions from doctors: "The problem is shortage of doctors and its ultimate aim must be to produce more doctors. We should face the problems squarely and solve it." Quoted in O. O. Akinkugbe et al. (eds.) *Priorities in National Health Planning* (Ibadan: Spectrum Books, 1981). Also, see S. O. Alubo, "The Political Economy of Doctors' Strikes in Nigeria: a Marxist Interpretation," *Social Science and Medicine* 22 (1986): 467-79.

37. "Nigeria's medical education system, well regarded by foreign authorities, is being expanded. Marketing executives will watch this development since the installation of advanced medical equipment in schools and universities is important for follow-on sales to health care establishments." From U.S. Department of Commerce, *Nigeria: a Survey of U.S. Business Opportunities* (Washington: Government Printing Office, 1976), p. 74.

38. Mburu, "Rhetoric Implementation."

39. A. Battersby, "Planning Health Services in Nigeria," *Disasters* 3 (1979): 179-83.

40. R. Stock, "Health Care for Some: a Nigerian Study of Who Gets What, Where and Why," *International Journal of Health Services* 15 (1985): 469-84.

41. *New Nigerian* (Kaduna), April 24, 1980.

42. Stock, "Health Care for Some."

43. World Health Organization, *Financing of Health Services* (Geneva: World Health Organization, 1978), pp. 94-101.

44. G. M. Mwabu and W. M. Mwangi, "Health Care Financing in Kenya: a Simulation of Welfare Effects of User Fees," *Social Science and Medicine* 22 (1986): 763-68. Also Mburu, "Rhetoric Implementation."

45. D. de Ferranti, *Paying for Health Services in Developing Countries: an Overview*, working paper no. 721 (Washington: World Bank, 1985); P. Musgrove, "What Should Consumers in Poor Countries Pay for Publicly-Provided Health Services?" *Social Science and Medicine* 22 (1986): 329-34.

46. S. O. Alubo, "Power and Privileges in Medical Care: an Analysis of Medical Services in Post-Colonial Nigeria," *Social Science and Medicine* 24 (1987): 453-62.
47. "Lambo hits at health treatments abroad," *West Africa*, March 5, 1984.
48. Alubo, "Political Economy of Doctors."
49. Young, *Ideology and Development*, p. 12.
50. P. J. Freund, "Health Care in a Declining Economy: the Case of Zambia," *Social Science and Medicine* 23 (1986).
51. T. A. Aidoo, "Rural Health Under Colonization and Neocolonization: A Survey of the Chadian Experience," *International Journal of Health Services* 12 (1982): 637-57; A. Beck, *Medicine, Tradition and Development in Kenya and Tanzania, 1920-1970* (Waltham, Mass.: Crossroads, 1981); D. E. Ferguson, "The Political Economy of Health and Medicine in Colonial Tanganyika," in *Tanzania Under Colonial Rule*, ed. M. H. Y. Kaniki (London: Longman, 1975), pp. 307-43.
52. Callaghy, "Difficulties."
53. P. J. Freund, "Health Care."
54. P. A. Maro, "Reducing Inequalities in the Distribution of Health Facilities in Tanzania," in *Health and Disease in Africa: Geographical and Medical Viewpoints*, ed. R. Akhtar (London: Harwood, 1987), pp. 415-27.
55. C. A. Anyinam, "Persistence with Change: A Rural-Urban Study of Ethno-Medical Practices in Contemporary Ghana," Ph.D. Diss., Department of Geography, Queen's University, 1987.
56. On Tanzania, see Beck, *Medicine*. On Zambia, see *Report of the First National Workshop on Traditional Medicine and its Role in the Development of Primary Health Care in Zambia* (Lusaka: Ministry of Health, 1977).
57. J. Nyerere, *Freedom and Socialism* (New York: Oxford, 1968).
58. W. K. Chagula and E. Tarimo, "Meeting Basic Health Needs in Tanzania," in *Health by the People*, ed. K. Newell (Geneva: World Health Organization, 1975), pp. 145-68; H. K. Heggenhougen, "Will Primary Health Care Efforts be Allowed to Succeed?" *Social Science and Medicine* 19 (1984): 217-24.

59. C. G. Kahama, T. L. Maliyamkono, and S. Wells, *The Challenge for Tanzania's Economy* (London: James Currey, 1986), pp. 163-75.

60. Heggenhougen, "Will Primary Health Care."

61. P. A. Twumasi and P. J. Freund, "Local Politicization of Primary Health Care as an Instrument for Development: A Case Study of Community Health Workers in Zambia," *Social Science and Medicine* 20 (1985): 1073-80.

62. Kahama et al., *The Challenge*, p. 171.

63. Kahama et al., *The Challenge*, p. 174.

64. Freund, "Health Care," p. 877.

65. Freund, "Health Care," p. 878-79.

66. Freund, "Health Care," p. 880.

67. C. A. Anyinam, "The Rawlings' Revolution and Primary Health Care in Ghana: An Assessment," paper presented at Canadian African Studies Association Conference, Kingston, Ontario, 1988.

68. A. I. Schoenholtz, "The IMF in Africa: Unnecessary and Undesirable Restraint on Western Development," *Journal of Modern African Studies* 25 (1987): 403-33.

69. K. Nkrumah, *Neocolonialism: The Last Stage of Imperialism* (London: Nelson, 1965).

70. Young, *Ideology and Development*, p. 12.

71. L. Rudebeck, *Guinea-Bissau: A Study of Political Mobilization* (Uppsala: Scandinavian Institute of African Studies, 1979), p. 199.

72. Rudebeck, *Guinea-Bissau*.

73. J. Hanlon, *Mozambique: The Revolution Under Fire* (London: Zed, 1984), p. 57.

74. Hanlon, *Mozambique*, pp. 65-71.

75. Hanlon, *Mozambique*, p. 56.

76. Hanlon, *Mozambique*, p. 58.

77. R. E. Galli and J. Jones, *Guinea-Bissau Politics, Economics and Society* (London: Frances Pinter, 1987).

78. Hanlon, *Mozambique*, p. 71.

79. D. Jelley and R. J. Madeley, "Primary Health Care in Practice: A Study in Mozambique," *Social Science and Medicine* 19 (1984): 773-80.

80. Hanlon, *Mozambique*, p. 62.

81. O. Gish, "Some Observations About Health Development in Three African Socialist Countries: Ethiopia, Mozambique and Tanzania," *Social Science and Medicine* 17 (1983): 1968.
82. Galli and Jones, *Guinea-Bissau*, pp. 183-84.
83. G. Bloom, "Two Models for Change in the Health Services in Zimbabwe," *International Journal of Health Services* 15 (1985): 451-68.
84. Bloom, "Two Models."
85. S. Decalo, "Ideological Rhetoric and Scientific Socialism in Benin and Congo/Brazzaville," in *Socialism in Sub-Saharan Africa: A New Assessment*, ed. C. G. Rosberg and T. M. Callaghy (Berkeley: Institute of International Studies, University of California, 1979), pp. 231-63.
86. Aidoo, "Rural Health."

MONOGRAPHS IN INTERNATIONAL STUDIES

ISBN Prefix 0-89680-

Africa Series

36. Fadiman, Jeffrey A. *The Moment of Conquest: Meru, Kenya, 1907.* 1979. 70pp.
    081-4 $ 5.50*

37. Wright, Donald R. *Oral Traditions From The Gambia: Volume I, Mandinka Griots.* 1979. 176pp.
    083-0 $15.00*

38. Wright, Donald R. *Oral Traditions From The Gambia: Volume II, Family Elders.* 1980. 200pp.
    084-9 $15.00*

41. Lindfors, Bernth. *Mazungumzo: Interviews with East African Writers, Publishers, Editors, and Scholars.* 1981. 179pp.
    108-X $13.00*

43. Harik, Elsa M. and Donald G. Schilling. *The Politics of Education in Colonial Algeria and Kenya.* 1984. 102pp.
    117-9 $12.50*

44. Smith, Daniel R. *The Influence of the Fabian Colonial Bureau on the Independence Movement in Tanganyika.* 1985. x, 98pp.
    125-X $11.00*

45. Keto, C. Tsehloane. *American-South African Relations 1784-1980: Review and Select Bibliography.* 1985. 159pp.
    128-4 $11.00*

46. Burness, Don, and Mary-Lou Burness, ed. *Wanasema: Conversations with African Writers*. 1985. 95pp.
129-2 $11.00*

47. Switzer, Les. *Media and Dependency in South Africa: A Case Study of the Press and the Ciskei "Homeland"*. 1985. 80pp.
130-6 $10.00*

48. Heggoy, Alf Andrew. *The French Conquest of Algiers, 1830: An Algerian Oral Tradition*. 1986. 101pp.
131-4 $11.00*

49. Hart, Ursula Kingsmill. *Two Ladies of Colonial Algeria: The Lives and Times of Aurelie Picard and Isabelle Eberhardt*. 1987. 156pp.
143-8 $11.00*

50. Voeltz, Richard A. *German Colonialism and the South West Africa Company, 1894-1914*. 1988. 143pp.
146-2 $12.00*

51. Clayton, Anthony, and David Killingray. *Khaki and Blue: Military and Police in British Colonial Africa*. 1989. 235pp.
147-0 $18.00*

52. Northrup, David. *Beyond the Bend in the River: African Labor in Eastern Zaire, 1865-1940*. 1988. 195pp.
151-9 $15.00*

53. Makinde, M. Akin. *African Philosophy, Culture, and Traditional Medicine*. 1988. 175pp.
152-7 $13.00*

54. Parson, Jack, ed. *Succession to High Office in Botswana. Three Case Studies*. 1990. 443pp.
157-8 $20.00*

55. Burness, Don. *A Horse of White Clouds*. 1989. 193pp.
158-6 $12.00*

56. Staudinger, Paul. *In the Heart of the Hausa States.* Tr. by Johanna Moody. 1990. 2 vols. 653pp.
160-8 $35.00*

57. Sikainga, Ahmad Alawad. *The Western Bahr Al-Ghazal Under British Rule: 1898-1956.* 1991. 183pp.
161-6 $15.00*

58. Wilson, Louis E. *The Krobo People of Ghana to 1892: A Political and Social History.* 1991. 254pp.
164-0 $20.00*

59. du Toit, Brian M. *Cannabis, Alcohol, and the South African Student: Adolescent Drug Use 1974-1985.* 1991. 166pp.
166-7 $17.00*

60. Falola, Toyin, ed. *The Political Economy of Health in Africa.* 1992. 254pp.
168-3 $17.00*

Latin America Series

8. Clayton, Lawrence A. *Caulkers and Carpenters in a New World: The Shipyards of Colonial Guayaquil.* 1980. 189pp, illus.
103-9 $15.00*

9. Tata, Robert J. *Structural Changes in Puerto Rico's Economy: 1947-1976.* 1981. xiv, 104pp.
107-1 $12.00*

11. O'Shaughnessy, Laura N., and Louis H. Serra. *Church and Revolution in Nicaragua.* 1986. 118pp.
126-8 $12.00*

12. Wallace, Brian. *Ownership and Development: A Comparison of Domestic and Foreign Investment in Colombian Manufacturing.* 1987. 186pp.
145-4 $10.00*

13. Henderson, James D. *Conservative Thought in Latin America: The Ideas of Laureano Gomez.* 1988. 150pp.
148-9 $13.00*

14. Summ, G. Harvey, and Tom Kelly. *The Good Neighbors: America, Panama, and the 1977 Canal Treaties.* 1988. 135pp.
149-7 $13.00*

15. Peritore, Patrick. *Socialism, Communism, and Liberation Theology in Brazil: An Opinion Survey Using Q-Methodology.* 1990. 245pp.
156-X $15.00*

16. Alexander, Robert J. *Juscelino Kubitschek and the Development of Brazil.* 1991. 429pp.
163-2 $25.00*

17. Mijeski, Kenneth J., ed. *The Nicaraguan Constitution of 1987: English Translation and Commentary.* 1990. 355pp.
165-9 $25.00*

Southeast Asia Series

31. Nash, Manning. *Peasant Citizens: Politics, Religion, and Modernization in Kelantan, Malaysia.* 1974. 181pp.
018-0 $12.00*

38. Bailey, Conner. *Broker, Mediator, Patron, and Kinsman: An Historical Analysis of Key Leadership Roles in a Rural Malaysian District.* 1976. 79pp.
024-5 $ 8.00*

44. Collier, William L., et al. *Income, Employment and Food Systems in Javanese Coastal Villages.* 1977. 160pp.
031-8 $10.00*

45. Chew, Sock Foon and MacDougall, John A. *Forever Plural: The Perception and Practice of Inter-Communal Marriage in Singapore.* 1977. 61pp.
030-X $ 8.00*

47. Wessing, Robert. *Cosmology and Social Behavior in a West Javanese Settlement.* 1978. 200pp.
072-5 $12.00*

48. Willer, Thomas F., ed. *Southeast Asian References in the British Parliamentary Papers, 1801-1972/73: An Index.* 1978. 110pp.
033-4 $ 8.50*

49. Durrenberger, E. Paul. *Agricultural Production and Household Budgets in a Shan Peasant Village in Northwestern Thailand: A Quantitative Description.* 1978. 142pp.
071-7 $10.00*

50. Echauz, Robustiano. *Sketches of the Island of Negros.* 1978. 174pp.
070-9 $12.00*

51. Krannich, Ronald L. *Mayors and Managers in Thailand: The Struggle for Political Life in Administrative Settings.* 1978. 139pp.
073-3 $11.00*

56A. Duiker, William J. *Vietnam Since the Fall of Saigon.* Updated edition. 1989. 383pp.
162-4 $17.00*

59. Foster, Brian L. *Commerce and Ethnic Differences: The Case of the Mons in Thailand.* 1982. x, 93pp.
112-8 $10.00*

60. Frederick, William H., and John H. McGlynn. *Reflections on Rebellion: Stories from the Indonesian Upheavals of 1948 and 1965.* 1983. vi, 168pp.
111-X $ 9.00*

61. Cady, John F. *Contacts With Burma, 1935-1949: A Personal Account.* 1983. x, 117pp.
114-4 $ 9.00*

63. Carstens, Sharon, ed. *Cultural Identity in Northern Peninsular Malaysia.* 1986. 91pp.
116-0 $ 9.00*

64. Dardjowidjojo, Soenjono. *Vocabulary Building in Indonesian: An Advanced Reader.* 1984. xviii, 256pp.
118-7 $26.00*

65. Errington, J. Joseph. *Language and Social Change in Java: Linguistic Reflexes of Modernization in a Traditional Royal Polity.* 1985. xiv, 211pp.
120-9 $20.00*

66. Binh, Tran Tu. *The Red Earth: A Vietnamese Memoir of Life on a Colonial Rubber Plantation.* Tr. by John Spragens. Ed. by David Marr. 1985. xii, 98pp.
119-5 $11.00*

68. Syukri, Ibrahim. *History of the Malay Kingdom of Patani.* Tr. by Conner Bailey and John N. Miksic. 1985. xix, 113pp.
123-3 $12.00*

69. Keeler, Ward. *Javanese: A Cultural Approach.* 1984. xxxvi, 523pp.
121-7 $18.00*

70. Wilson, Constance M., and Lucien M. Hanks. *Burma-Thailand Frontier Over Sixteen Decades: Three Descriptive Documents.* 1985. x, 128pp.
124-1 $11.00*

71. Thomas, Lynn L., and Franz von Benda-Beckmann, eds. *Change and Continuity in Minangkabau: Local, Regional, and Historical Perspectives on West Sumatra.* 1986. 363pp.
127-6 $16.00*

72. Reid, Anthony, and Oki Akira, eds. *The Japanese Experience in Indonesia: Selected Memoirs of 1942-1945.* 1986. 411pp., 20 illus.
132-2 $20.00*

73. Smirenskaia, Zhanna D. *Peasants in Asia: Social Consciousness and Social Struggle.* Tr. by Michael J. Buckley. 1987. 248pp.
134-9 $14.00

74. McArthur, M.S.H. *Report on Brunei in 1904.* Ed. by A.V.M. Horton. 1987. 304pp.
135-7 $15.00

75. Lockard, Craig Alan. *From Kampung to City. A Social History of Kuching Malaysia 1820-1970.* 1987. 311pp.
136-5 $16.00*

76. McGinn, Richard. *Studies in Austronesian Linguistics.* 1988. 492pp.
137-3 $20.00*

77. Muego, Benjamin N. *Spectator Society: The Philippines Under Martial Rule.* 1988. 232pp.
138-1 $15.00*

78. Chew, Sock Foon. *Ethnicity and Nationality in Singapore.* 1987. 229pp.
139-X $12.50*

79. Walton, Susan Pratt. *Mode in Javanese Music.* 1987. 279pp.
144-6 $15.00*

80. Nguyen Anh Tuan. *South Vietnam Trial and Experience: A Challenge for Development.* 1987. 482pp.
141-1 $18.00*

81. Van der Veur, Paul W., ed. *Toward a Glorious Indonesia: Reminiscences and Observations of Dr. Soetomo.* 1987. 367pp.
142-X $16.00*

82. Spores, John C. *Running Amok: An Historical Inquiry.* 1988. 190pp.
140-3 $14.00*

83. Tan Malaka. *From Jail to Jail.* Tr. and ed. by Helen Jarvis. 1990. 3 vols. 1,226pp.
150-0 $55.00*

84. Devas, Nick. *Financing Local Government in Indonesia.* 1989. 344pp.
153-5 $16.00*

85. Suryadinata, Leo. *Military Ascendancy and Political Culture: A Study of Indonesia's Golkar.* 1989. 222pp.
179-9 $15.00*

86. Williams, Michael. *Communism, Religion, and Revolt in Banten.* 1990. 356pp.
155-1 $16.00*

87. Hudak, Thomas John. *The Indigenization of Pali Meters in Thai Poetry.* 1990. 237pp.
159-4 $15.00*

88. Lay, Ma Ma. *Not Out of Hate: A Novel of Burma.* Tr. by Margaret Aung-Thwin. Ed. by William Frederick. 1991. 222pp.
167-5 $20.00*

ORDERING INFORMATION

Orders for titles in the Monographs in International Studies series may be placed through the Ohio University Press, Scott Quadrangle, Athens, Ohio 45701-2979 or through any local bookstore. Individuals should remit payment by check, VISA, MasterCard, or American Express. People ordering from the United Kingdom, Continental Europe, the Middle East, and Africa should order through Academic and University Publishers Group, 1 Gower Street, London WC1E, England. Orders from the Pacific Region, Asia, Australia, and New Zealand should be sent to East-West Export Books, c/o the University of Hawaii Press, 2840 Kolowalu Street, Honolulu, Hawaii 96822, USA.

Other individuals ordering from outside of the U.S. should remit in U.S. funds to the Ohio University Press either by International Money Order or by a check drawn on a U.S. bank. Most out-of-print titles may be ordered from University Microfilms, Inc., 300 North Zeeb Road, Ann Arbor, Michigan 48106, USA.

Prices do not include shipping charges and are subject to change without notice.